CONTENTS

KV-019-565

SUMMARY

The findings of a two-year research project are reported. The study examines, from the patients' perspective, aspects of the doctor/patient relationship with regard to general practice.

Two general practitioners co-operated in the study, and 320 of their patients. The sample was drawn by random method in two groups: the first group was interviewed at the practice prior to consulting the doctor, and again at their own homes; the second group was contacted by letter and respondents were interviewed once at home. Semi-structured questionnaires were used and the doctors contributed secondary data by completing a record form of the relevant consultations. All consultations in the study period were recorded on audiotape, with the permission of the patients. Only those consultations relating to the study were retained.

The method and problems of carrying out a study of this nature are examined.

The interaction between doctor and patient begins effectively with the reception of the latter at the practice. Two different systems of receiving patients are assessed. The role of the doctors' receptionists as a funnel or filter is discussed. Whilst patients accept the receptionist's function as manager of the practice's appointments system, they are likely to regard her assessment of priority of need for a visit or appointment with resentment. Such assessment and advice would be readily accepted from a general practice nurse. There seems little doubt that a formal course of training for receptionists, which included an appropriate level of medical competence and elements of the behavioural sciences, would benefit both patients and receptionists.

Patients' views of "personal doctoring" are assessed by their attitudes towards continuity of care, the presence of a third party in the consultation, and the doctors' role of general adviser and confidante. As a further indicator, their preferences for personal or impersonal styles of doctor/patient communication are assessed. Analysis of the data shows that the doctors' role as friend of the family is likely to be the desirable ideal of the profession itself, but is not reciprocated by the patient. Pastoral interest on the part of the doctor was most likely to be rejected by his social and educational peers, and by the younger patients. Objectivity on the part of the doctor, coupled with a friendly but business-like approach appeared to be more appreciated by the patients than personal aspects of the relationship.

Interaction of patients' expectations and the fulfilment of these in the consultation is examined with regard to the five most commonly occurring actions taken in the doctor's management of patients. These are: issuing certificates for national insurance benefits (sick notes), prescribing, examining patients, arranging investigations and arranging referrals. Satisfaction or dissatisfaction with the consultation was not necessarily dependent upon the outcome of pre-consultation expectations *per se*, but was determined by the strength of these expectations.

The quality of communication between doctor and patient and the expectations attached to their interacting roles are found to be essential factors in determining whether patients express their needs and expectations. Specific barriers to communication in the consultation are identified. From the patients' perspective, these most often emanated from the doctor. In the prevailing climate of doctor/patient interaction, the patient is generally vulnerable and often anxious. Conditions which produce the minimum of anxiety in the consultation would inevitably facilitate communication and thereby promote the common interests of both doctor and patient, i.e. the patient's return to health or optimum capacity. Awareness of their patients' perspective may be best acquired through application by general practitioners of the behavioural sciences.

F.F.
H.W.K.A.

PREFACE

When patients seek advice on health matters their expectations will depend upon their perception of the role of the person from whom they seek advice. Advice may be sought from various sources, including friends, relatives and neighbours, as well as professional health advisers. Patients' perception of the role of available advisers will be dependent upon their experience of the success or otherwise of previous encounters, the reported experience of others and the attitudes engendered by descriptive statements emanating from official and unofficial sources and from general hearsay.

No matter from whom advice is sought, the process begins with a patient's description of the problem and normally ends with the receipt of advice. In short, a consultation takes place. In medical practice it is from the consultation that all medical care is derived.

The dynamics of the consultation depend upon many factors, including the competence of the adviser and the framework within which patient and adviser are operating. The interaction between them becomes a complex of ethical, cultural and personal factors. Examination of the consultation between doctor and patient is therefore a study in human behaviour which must be based upon human behaviour as it is and not as we want it to be.[1]

In the National Health Service general practitioners contract to provide services. Two types of contract are involved: an explicit contract with the Family Practitioner Committee acting as agent for the Department of Health and Social Security; and an implicit contract with the patient. In mounting this study our objective was to examine some aspects of the implicit contract, in particular the expectations and requirements which patients have in mind when they come to consult a general practitioner and whether these are fulfilled.

The fulfilment of patients' expectations and requirements will depend upon the effectiveness of communication between patient and doctor, the validity of the patient's expectations and the ability of the doctor to fulfil them or, if he is unable to do so, to make an appropriate referral.

The principles of communication have been stated to be:[2]

1 The purpose of communication is not just to deliver a message but to effect a change in the recipient in respect of his knowledge, his attitude or, eventually, in his behaviour.

2 The value of a communication is to be judged not on its purpose or content but on its effect on the recipient. An elegant or witty communication may satisfy the communicator but leave the recipient uninformed and unmoved.

3 Good communication is difficult. Few can master it without special tuition and constant attention to its effectiveness.

4 The occasion must be matched to the knowledge, initial background, interests, purposes, and needs of the recipient. It requires empathy which is "the power of projecting one's personality into, and so fully understanding, the object of contemplation".

5 Communication is effected not only by words which must have the same meaning for giver and receiver, but also by attitudes, expressions and

gestures. This is especially relevant to a consultation where patient and doctor are both givers and receivers.

6 If the communication is to change behaviour, the required change in the recipient must be seen by him to have more advantages than drawbacks; otherwise it will not be made, or if it is made, will not persist. New information resulting in a change of attitude is usually a necessary prelude to a change in behaviour.

7 To make sure that a communication has succeeded, information about its effects ('feedback') both immediate or subsequent is needed.

8 Communication demands effort, thought, time, and often money. Effective communication between colleagues also demands willingness on the part of the giver to discover that more may be learnt than taught.

As Professor Fletcher points out, there is virtually no medical activity which does not involve communication.

The effectiveness, or otherwise, of communication figures largely in the results of our study, which also cast some light upon attitudes and how they may be perceived by both patient and doctor.

Many of the opinions concerning the relationship between general practitioners and their patients emanate from general practitioners themselves and are, therefore, subject to bias. This study was initiated by a general practitioner who was well aware of this possibility. The construction of the questionnaires, the interviewing of patients and the interpretation of the data were, by design, carried out by persons who had received no medical training whatsoever, and doctor orientated bias has been eliminated as far as possible.

Patients' expectations are relevant to the need to balance "wants" with "needs" and the resources available. The Royal College of General Practitioners[3] put forward five questions:

1 Who is best able to provide care?
2 What care is it useful to provide?
3 Where is care best given?
4 When should care be given and what length of delays are intolerable?
5 Why is the care being given, how and with what results?

It is upon such questions as these that the whole organization of medical care depends. They can never be answered irrevocably because answers will change as resources change, and as medical or social priorities alter. The last of these five questions is the most important and it was for this reason that we began our inquiry into the process of care in general practice at the point where the patient has decided to seek medical advice, and to determine the extent to which the patient, as customer, believes that his requirements are being met.

H.W.K.A.
F.F.

REFERENCES

1. Bloom, S. W. (1963). *The Doctor and His Patient.* New York: Russell Sage Foundation.

2. Fletcher, C. M. (1973). *Communication in Medicine.* London: The Nuffield Provincial Hospitals Trust.

3. Royal College of General Practitioners (1973). "Present State and Future Needs of General Practice." Report from General Practice No. 16, *Journal of the Royal College of General Practitioners.*

ACKNOWLEDGEMENTS

We are deeply grateful to the Department of Health and Social Security who provided the funds for this study and to Professor Gordon Forsyth whose advice and encouragement was of immense value throughout. We are indebted to Miss Peggy Foster who shared in the organization of the research, the construction of the questionnaires and the interviewing of respondents and to Neil Fitton for his encouragement and constructive criticism.

We wish to record our immense gratitude to the general practitioner colleagues who allowed their patients to be interviewed and to the staff of their practices. Without their co-operation the study could not have been carried out.

To Miss Joan Bowker and others who shared the secretarial work we convey our grateful thanks for their manifold assistance.

Finally, we wish to thank all the patients who took part in the study for their co-operation, and on many occasions their hospitality, often at some inconvenience to themselves and their families, and the many colleagues and friends who helped us to explore the avenues of doctor/patient interaction in general practice.

F.F.
H.W.K.A.

CHAPTER I
INTRODUCTION

Theoretical approaches to the sociological analysis of the doctor/patient relationship embrace a broad spectrum derived mainly from Parsons' concept of the complementary roles of doctor and patient set in the context of social systems maintenance in modern industrial societies.[1,2] Integral to this approach is the concept of role theory.

Role theory

Role theory utilizes the drama analogy and is based on the model of man as an actor, whose behaviour is modified and internalized in accordance with the commonly perceived action expectations related to the part being played; in this case that of doctor and patient. These expectations enhance the probability that in a given social situation individuals will act to a great extent in a pre-determined manner.

Parsons' concern is not with analyzing the range of behaviour relating to interaction in the doctor/patient relationship but in the construction of an ideal type of abstract generality as formulated in Weber's analysis. The ideal type is " . . . an ideal construction of a typical course of action, or form of relationship, which is applicable to the analysis of an indefinable plurality of concrete cases and which formulates in pure, logically consistent form certain elements that are relevant to the understanding of the several concrete situations."[3]

This abstraction represents the essential elements of a phenomenon in a pure form which rarely, if ever, occurs. The term "ideal" is not used in the normative or exemplary sense, implying that realization is desirable, but in the logical sense as a heuristic device. The pure type provides a yardstick by which to measure, assess and explain deviation in the concrete case.[4]

In his structural-functionalist model Parsons treats illness as dysfunctional and deviant, in that by becoming sick the individual fails to fulfil expectations attached to his role in the social system.

Illness is not only a condition but also a social role, with attached expectations of appropriate behaviour. The sick role incumbent is not held by society to be responsible for his condition and is exempt from normal social obligations in accordance with the severity of his illness. The patient is obliged to gain legitimation for his status by accepted, generalized, objective criteria, and to seek technically competent aid; he is expected to co-operate fully in his desire to become well and to become fully reintegrated into the social system. Bloor and Horobin[5] take issue with Parsons in his elementary failure to distinguish conceptually between the sick role and the patient role. Persons may successfully claim the sick role without seeking professional aid and, alternatively, may accept treatment as a patient without expecting or receiving exemption from social obligations.

In Parsons' model the complementary role of the physician is functionally specific, in that the basis of competence is related to expertise in a specialized field and not to "generalized wisdom". The acceptance by the patient of the physician's interpretation of his illness is based upon the latter's validated technical competence and the prestige attached by society to his scientific training.

The primary orientation of the physician is to the welfare of the patient with the exclusion of the profit motive. Parsons distinguishes two aspects of medical practice: the instrumental function dealing with technical matters, and the expressive function concerning psychological and social factors. Parsons refers to the latter as the "art of medicine", which he contends is a major part of the skilful practice of medicine.

Special informal and formal features are built into the role expectations of the doctor/patient dyad as a protective mechanism in relation to the unavoidably intimate nature of the relationship. These include the confidentiality of the consultation and medical records, and strict control of the use of information given by patients. The ethics of the medical profession prohibit the intrusion into the consultation of any sexual relationship, the most severe sanctions being attached to any departure from this principle. The doctor's approach is affectively neutral in that he is not affected by like or dislike of the patient, nor by the patient's aggression or attachment to him. His function is that of an objective scientist whose concern is limited to matters of health.

In Parsons' model the roles of the sick patient and the physician are complementary in relation to shared values and expectations and to the maintenance of the social system. However, they are not reciprocal in terms of emotional and general social intercourse. The patient may regard the doctor as a friend and confidante, revealing his most private life and fears, whilst a return of such intimacy would be entirely inappropriate. Additional significance is attached to the role of the physician in that by facilitating the social reintegration of his patient he stands at a strategic position in the maintenance of the equilibrium of the social system.

The psychoanalytic approach

Parsons' model and the psychoanalytic approach to analysis of the doctor/patient relationship are both contrasting and complementary. In general terms, Parsons perceives illness as a deviant position in the social structure, the incidence of which needs to be controlled constantly by another social group, the medical profession.

The psychoanalytic approach regards illness as a process affecting the individual. The patient is viewed as a person who requires the help of the physician in a co-operative endeavour which seeks to unravel the special, specific social causes which have brought him to illness.

The two approaches are closely connected and complementary in that, by definition, illness is concerned with physical, psychological and social aspects and elements of motivation towards deviance.

Parsons maintains that all good medical practice contains a degree of psychotherapy. Whether deliberately or unconsciously applied, this is a feature of the doctor's role in its particular meshing with the sick role. As a mechanism of social control the sick role provides a legitimate channel in which deviance engendered by social strain and regressive tendencies can be given expression under appropriate cover. Motivation for the sick role may also involve secondary gain which the patient, consciously or unconsciously, wishes to secure. In fact the problem for the doctor may be first to determine the deeper psychological problem underlying the physical symptoms "offered" by the patient.

10

Yudkin[6] refers to this aspect as the "second diagnosis", which may place greater demands on the doctor's diagnostic and therapeutic skills.

Balint[7] points out that it is much easier for patients to approach the doctor with a physical symptom rather than with the cause of underlying anxiety which they may find difficult to define and to express verbally. The physical symptoms offered to the doctor may have little relevance to the real reason for attending which may be veiled to a varying degree. The elucidation of the underlying problem will be dependent upon the doctor's perception and interpretation of offered "hints".

Far from being a process of openly expressed expectations and exchange of information, communication between doctor and patient is based on the strategic selection of offered information, consciously or unconsciously sifted. The covert content of the consultation may be of considerable significance to both doctor and patient but remain unexpressed or only barely hinted at. Unless the doctor has well developed powers of interpretation and perception and is motivated to use these skills to arrive at a deeper diagnosis, the underlying state of anxiety may assume greater proportions than the original problem. Direct close questioning by the doctor is, according to Balint, entirely futile: "Our experience has been that, if the doctor asks questions in the manner of medical history taking he will always get answers—but hardly anything more."[7, p.121] Many doctors may choose to hear "nothing more", preferring the non-involvement of a technocratic encounter that leaves feelings out of the consultation.

Balint differentiates between "illness-centred medicine", which involves the doctor's active concentration on the physical treatment in a brief consultation, and "patient-orientated medicine". The latter may involve lengthy interviews, with patient and doctor seeking together to unravel cause and effect. This technique is more applicable to the practice of psychotherapy than general practice. In recognition of this, Balint initiated research into short-term therapy. The results[8] appeared to confirm that the principles of psychotherapy can be utilized effectively in the context of the concentrated interview appropriate to general practice. By developing finely tuned perception, the doctor is able to recognize the "flash point" in the consultation; that is, the moment when the patient reveals what really is troubling him.

The two styles of illness-centred medicine and patient-centred medicine are not mutually exclusive in one practitioner. For example, a practitioner who is consistently more interested in patients' illnesses derived from the stresses of alcoholism, may set aside his normal pattern of practising illness-centred medicine when presented with such patients. However, the general style adopted by a doctor may become fixed by constant repetition so that patients come to be educated not only in the general role expectations of the doctor/patient relationhip but in the finer tuning of their expected behaviour in regard to a particular doctor.

In their path-finding study of the verbal behaviour of general practitioners, Byrne and Long,[9, p.8] comment upon their observations of 103 doctors that, " . . . older practitioners had learned particular patterns of consulting in which even the way they asked questions had become stereotyped". Their impression is one of doctors so set in their ways that patient behaviour is irrelevant. Balint[7, p.216] contends that doctors have firmly conditioned patients'

11

expectations of how they should behave: "It was almost as if every doctor had revealed knowledge of what was right and what was wrong for patients to expect and endure and, further, as if he had a sacred duty to convert to his faith all the ignorant and unbelieving among his patients." Centred around this "apostolic function" are a host of expectations and proscriptions which regulate patients' behaviour and communication in the consultation, according to the habitual behaviour of the doctor rather than the patient.

The "apostolic function" also takes the form of the administration of "self". Balint contends that the doctor himself is the most potent "drug" which he prescribes, whether this be as authoritative guardian, detached scientist, protective parent or trusted adviser in an equal partnership.

There is little doubt that a relationship based on equality requires not only more giving on the part of the doctor, but his relinquishment of superior power in the dyad.

The power structure of the doctor/patient relationship

Analyses of the power structure of the doctor/patient relationship show clearly that although in terms of social-system maintenance the roles may be reciprocal, the dyad is inherently one of inequality and conflict.

Szasz and Hollender[10] define three ideal type models of the structure relating to doctor/patient interaction. Each is associated with the technical procedures involved and relates consecutively to the prototype relationships of parent/infant, parent/child and adult/adult.

In the activity/passivity model the doctor is in complete control. Whatever takes place between doctor and patient cannot be described as interaction. The patient is not in a position to respond actively but is wholly submissive to the techniques applied. For the doctor, the anaesthetized or unconscious patient may present the ideal situation for the treatment of organic illness.

The guidance/co-operation model also places the doctor in a position of superior power over the consulting patient. Although both participants are active in that they contribute to the interaction, only the doctor is in possession of the technical knowledge and expertise to make clinical judgments and prescribe management programmes. He may also possess knowledge about the patient's condition which he considers it better not to reveal. The patient, in his subordinate position, is not required or expected to question the "doctor's orders" deemed to be necessary for his own good, but to co-operate fully in all judgments. The latent power of the doctor to exert control over the provision of strategic resources, such as documents supporting claims for social security benefit, creates additional pressure on the patient to co-operate.

The third model is one of mutual participation and maximum co-operation. This approach is appropriate in the management of chronic conditions in which the patient monitors his own treatment programme to a great extent, and to the management of psychological or social problems where the patient's insight contributes significantly. The doctor does not profess to know exactly what is best for the patient at all times and the patient is not expected, nor does he expect, to take a passive role. The two participants are involved in devizing a treatment programme which makes sense to both in practical and emotional terms, and which is directed towards the mutually desirable goal of returning the patient to health or optimum functioning. This is the ideal of equality in a

12

mature and democratic association which becomes most appropriate when the dyad consists of intellectual and social peers, but which it should be within the doctor's skill to apply to patients who are not his peers intellectually or socially.

Freidson[11] points out that a logical extension of the typology should include reversal of the doctor/patient roles in the guidance/co-operation and activity/passivity models. In reality, doctors often act in direct response to patients' requests for a prescription or referral. Duff and Hollingshead[12] also point out that the normative power structure in the relationship is reversed to a great degree when patients pay for their doctor's services. Patients are then in a stronger position to question the doctor's decisions, thus posing a threat to his authority. His income may also be threatened if he does not meet patients' demands. The failure of Szasz and Hollender to include Freidson's extension of the typology indicates a doctor-orientated perspective of the balance of power in the doctor/patient relationship.

In modern industrial societies there is little doubt that Szasz and Hollender's guidance/co-operation model prevails. The patient is, by definition, a layman in matters of health care considered appropriate to take to the doctor. As such, he is not in a position to assess the technical competence of the physician. In effect, he judges his condition from an entirely different perspective. The inevitable culture gap which is built into the sick-role model, then becomes a source of potential conflict, with the possibility of mistrust and dissatisfaction on both sides.

Freidson[13] contends that "... the separate worlds of experience and reference of the layman and the professional worker are always in potential conflict with each other. This seems to be inherent in the very situation of professional practice." Bloor and Horobin[5] elaborate further on the culture gap between professional and layman. Borrowing the term "double bind" from psychology, which describes a situation where contradictory meanings are communicated in the same environment resulting in emotional confusion for the individual, they refer to the double bind situation of the patient faced with inconsistency between his own definition of the situation and that of the doctor to whom he must defer.

The individual who has convinced significant others that he is ill and has gained emotional and practical concessions as a result, stands to lose face if the doctor subsequently pronounces that nothing is wrong. The degree of loss of face will correlate directly with the number and quality of concessions. If these are considerable, the patient may be unwilling to set aside his own definition of the situation and defer to that of the doctor. Criticism of the doctor's judgment is implicit in taking this option and may result in conflict between patient and doctor. The patient may then resort to "shopping around" in an attempt to seek a professional verdict which agrees with his own perception, or in overt acceptance of the doctor's judgment which is restricted to the consulting room.

This double bind situation also affects the relationship between doctor and patient from the doctor's perspective.

The patient who presents symptoms which can neither be observed nor accounted for must nevertheless be managed. If the doctor declares that he can find nothing wrong, he may be implying that the patient has consulted without reason. The patient may interpret this as an indication that the doctor considers him to be "neurotic". To avoid this effect, the doctor may prescribe a placebo

13

and/or ask the patient to return if the trouble does not clear up. The first option could reinforce for the patient the notion that something *was* wrong; the second risks damage to the doctor/patient relationship by placing the patient on the defensive. Deference on the part of the patient may often be more apparent then real, as shown by many studies of patients' compliance with doctors' instruction and advice.[14,15,16,17,18] These studies are generally to be found in the medical literature and, as such, present a view of the patient from the doctor's perspective. The terms used to refer to unco-operative patients (e.g. deviant, defaulter, non-compliant) reflect the position of the patient in the Parsonian model as passive; an obedient recipient in an unequal relationship dominated by the doctor.

Cultural aspects

Theorists seek to analyze the sick role as a social phenomenon in terms of the actual norms and attitudes of individuals and the cultural aspects surrounding their decision whether or not to seek professional aid.

Mechanic[19] contends that sickness is, in part, a subjective experience. The recognition of symptoms as worthy of action is determined in the context of norms which vary from one cultural group to another and one condition to another. Mechanic proposes the concept of "illness behaviour" which explains "...the ways in which given symptoms may be differentially perceived, evaluated and acted (or not acted) upon by different kinds of persons." Illness behaviour, in effect, determines whether diagnosis and treatment will be initiated at all. This theoretical approach is located firmly within a social action frame of reference. In accordance with Weber's theory[20] social actions of the individual are analyzed in terms of the meaning that the action holds for the actors, orientated to past, present or expected future behaviour of others in a social relationship.

Behaviour is related to the conscious choice of an active individual seeking to define the elements of his situation and synthesize these into an appropriate course of action. The decision whether or not to take action by seeking professional medical care may be determined by such factors as the strategic and economic importance of the individual's contribution to the family and work group, the ability to tolerate stress and discomfort, together with the culturally acquired perception and attitude towards these factors.

In his study of attitudes and action towards health care, Koos[14] found that the passage from tolerance of symptoms to seeking professional aid related to the individual's perception of discomfort and the implications upon his social position and life style of seeking professional advice. It appeared to be the cultural norm for older inhabitants of Regionville, in all social groups, to accept aches and pains as their lot in life and therefore hardly worthy of comment. Action decisions, including the decision to take no action, consistently related to an individual's location in the socio-economic structure. Lower social groups reported experiencing more symptoms than upper social groups but were less likely to see their doctor, especially if they provided the main source of income for the family. When economic considerations were not significant, the individual was more likely to consult a doctor. As one respondent said:[14, p.30]

> "Some people can be sick any time with anything, but most of us can't be sick, even when we need to be."

14

Although Koos' study describes the situation prevailing in the United States, it is also directly applicable to contemporary Britain. With employment figures currently in excess of $1\frac{1}{2}$ million and the prospects of redundancy a very real threat to many, it would not be expedient for insecure employees to ask for time off work in order to see their doctor.

The meaning attached to experience of discomfort is translated by the individual in terms of the likely effect upon his economic position of seeking medical advice. This commonsense theoretical interpretation of the empirical findings presupposes that the individual does not see himself as having a choice in course of action once he has initiated formal medical proceedings and is in receipt of doctor's orders. This implication is consistent with Parsons' model, which presents the doctors' view of an ideal, passive patient.

Zoborowski[21] analyzed the individual's interpretation and response to symptoms in four ethnic groups: Jewish, Italian, Irish and "Old American". The data showed clearly defined, consistent patterns of illness behaviour relating to each group.

The "Old Americans" showed most concern about the effect their illness might have in the future and were generally more optimistic about this than the Jewish Americans, who also tended to focus on the future. The Irish and the "Old Americans" were far more stoical in their response to pain and reported symptoms in what appeared to be an objective manner. Jewish patients tended to focus on the meaning of the symptom, and both Jews and Italians were very emotional in relating symptoms and tended to exaggerate them.

Distinguishing illness behaviour in relation to ethnic groups has also been studied by Zola[22] who asserts that illness behaviour cannot be understood without reference to the individual's cultural background and social environment for definition of the subjective meaning attached to perception of symptoms.

In an elegant and controlled study, Zola[22] analyzes the influence of ethnic group membership upon the selective process which determines whether or not to seek professional aid for relief of symptoms. The two groups studied were Irish Catholics and Italian Catholics, selected in pairs matched for disorder, degree of seriousness, duration, age, marital status and education. The empirical evidence relating to the Italians' attitude to illness supports that of Zoborowski. The Italians reported more symptoms and were far more emotional in describing discomfort and the effect this had on their life style. Also, they were more likely to stress related diffusion of a condition to other areas of the body. In considering the circumstances which led to seeking medical aid, they were more likely to have taken action on perceiving the effects of the illness on their social and personal relationships as significant.

In interpreting the data, the speculation is made that illness behaviour reflects major values determining formal and informal sanctions and attitudes towards handling problems. Zola refers to the "fit of certain bodily states with dominant value systems"[22, p.38] and makes the tentative supposition that the Italians' over-statement of symptoms is not only related to their general expansiveness but is a defence mechanism, a way of coping with anxiety by dissipating it. Their preferred method of handling the problem of anxiety contrasts with that of the Irish, who tended to ignore bodily complaints and understate symptoms as a defence mechanism. Zola contends that the illness

15

behaviour of each group is entirely consistent with their general view of life. The significant differences in the illness behaviour which emerged in the study correlated more consistently with ethnic group membership than any of the other demographic data taken into account.

In a further analysis of the data, Zola[23] explored the hypothesis that the manner in which the patient communicated a complaint to the doctor was directly related to the subsequent diagnosis. This appears to be confirmed by the evidence taken from a sub-group of patients who presented symptoms for which no organic basis was found. There was a statistically significant variation in diagnosis between the Irish and Italian patients, in that the Italians were far more likely to be assessed as having psychological problems. The diagnosis appeared to have been based entirely on non-medical factors but related to the way in which the patient communicated his condition to the doctor as a function of his singular perception of the problem.

The implications of these and other supportive findings for medical practice in Western societies which are rapidly becoming multi-racial, are obvious. The doctor's concept of what constitutes a "good patient" is likely to fit the norm of his own indigenous culture and his family, ethnic and ethical values, (Figure 1). Patient behaviour which does not accord with this stereotype may be met with at least suspicion and, at worst, disbelief on the part of the doctor, leading to inappropriate diagnosis. The therapeutic outcome of an encounter may never reach its potential unless the doctor is fully cognisant of the different patterns of illness behaviour relating to the individual's ethnic and cultural location in society.

Figure 1 Doctor/patient interaction

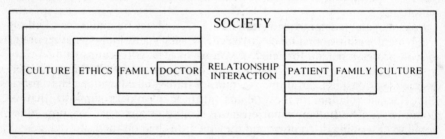

The patients' perspective

The foregoing theories and related empirical findings are concerned with the structure and function of the relationship between doctor and patient and, as such, provide the theoretical framework for analysis. However, they are not concerned with the actual content of interaction.

Byrne and Long[9, p.11] contend that as so little of the patient's verbal behaviour in the consultation can be viewed as "effect" it is almost irrelevant to what actually transpires during the consultation. For the purpose of erecting a typology of the verbal behaviour of consulting general practitioners for use as a tool in teaching communication skills, the approach is undoubtedly valid. Its value has been quickly realized by general practitioner trainees in many countries and utilized by general practitioners for a personal critical audit of their communication styles.

The effects of particular modes of communication may be a major factor in the quality of medical care. The study undertaken by Byrne and Long does not profess to assess the meaning of the doctor/patient interaction in terms of the reality for the patient. It does, however, take a narrow view of the consultation and reflects the Parsonian concept of the patient as a passive, compliant participant, whose moves in the consultation are almost entirely directed and restricted by the doctor. This view of the patient is reminiscent of Freud's concept of the emergent personality as yet unformed; an inactive, opinionless organism, moving at the mercy of significant others.

The relationship between doctor and patient does not exist in a consultation vacuum. To focus solely on the content of the consultation as a means of understanding the doctor/patient relationship may be to assign to it a disproportionate significance. Stimson and Webb[24] remind us that the face-to-face encounter is but one step in a social process which includes a host of related actions which take place in a wide social context before and after consultation. In this very perceptive study Stimson and Webb look at the doctor/patient relationship from the patient's perspective.

Using data collected from 96 patients consulting at two general practices and material from informal discussions in various other settings, Stimson and Webb analyze the consultation as a process set in the context of continuous social interaction rather than as an isolated incident. Although there are major areas of bias in the study, perhaps the most important is the unmethodical selection of respondents by practice receptionists, this does not detract from the sometimes startling degree of authenticity in the descriptive analysis. In his review of the study, Professor J. S. McCormick,[25] himself a general practitioner, maintains that, " . . . no practitioner could read this account without feeling that the perceptions of these patients are unlikely to be unusual and may be extremely widespread". Assessment of patients' attitudes in his own practice has accordingly been re-estimated without benefit of blinkers.

By illuminating patients' views from the "outside" the behavioural norms which form a barrier in the face-to-face interaction between doctor and patient are lowered. The general practitioner is presented with a more realistic view of his patients' perceptions of the consultation and the doctor/patient relationship in a wider context.

Taking an objective and practical approach, Ann Cartwright[26] has provided a wealth of invaluable, detailed information portraying the relationship between doctors and patients. Her large-scale study of the view of 1,397 respondents was drawn from the electoral registers of 12 areas in England and Wales, and included information on practice structure and general attitudes of the 422 general practitioners consulted by these respondents. The empirical findings form the basis of reported statistical data in a wide variety of studies and will be drawn upon widely by us.

In the study reported here, the views of 320 patients from two general practices form the main source of data. Secondary information has also been drawn from the two general practitioners concerned in relation to the specific condition or problem of consulting patients.

The theoretical orientation of the enquiry is located firmly in an approach which brings forward the patient as an active individual with definite views of his/her own position and the doctor's position. This approach does not represent an attempt to redress the balance of power in the dyad but rather to present the patient as a person, not as a problem or deviant member of society, as has been the general trend in theory and related research until quite recently. It is not the patient *per se* who is the subject of the study but the doctor, in the sense that we are looking at him from the patients' perspective in relation to a specific consultation and the wider context of the ongoing social relationship. Assessment of the quality of clinical care has no part in the study except insofar as this may be affected by the quality of the interaction between patient and doctor. By focusing on the meaning of the interaction from this "other side", we are attempting to contribute to a more balanced account of what transpires in the consultation and an essentially realistic picture of individuals' expectations in the context of primary medical care.

REFERENCES

1. Parsons, T. (1951). "Illness and the role of the Physician: a Sociological Perspective," *American Journal of Orthopsychiatry, 21,* 452.

2. Parsons, T. (1951). *The Social System.* London: Routledge and Kegan Paul.

3. Parsons, T. (1949). *The Structure of Social Action.* New York: The Free Press of Glencoe, p. 606.

4. Weber, M. (1964). *The Theory of Social and Economic Organisation.* Ed. with introduction by Parsons, T. New York: The Free Press of Glencoe.

5. Bloor, M. J. and Horobin, G. W. (1975). "Conflict and conflict resolution in doctor/patient interactions." In *A Sociology of Medical Practice.* Eds. Cox, A. and Mead, A. London: Collier-Macmillan.

6. Yudkin, S. (1961). "Six children with coughs—the second diagnosis," *Lancet ii,* 561.

7. Balint, M. (1964). *The Doctor, His Patient and the Illness.* London: Pitman Medical.

8. Balint, E. and Norell, J. S. Eds. (1973). "Six Minutes for the Patient: interactions in general practice consultations," *Mind and Medicine Monographs* No. 23. London: Tavistock Press.

9. Byrne, P. S. and Long, B. E. L. (1976). *Doctors Talking to Patients.* London: H.M.S.O.

10. Szasz, T. and Hollender, M. H. (1956). "A contribution to the Philosophy of Medicine," *Archives of Internal Medicine, 97,* 585.

11. Freidson, E. (1970). *Profession of Medicine.* New York: Dodds Mead and Co.

12. Duff, S. and Hollingshead, A. B. (1968). *Sickness and Society.* New York: Harper and Row.

13. Freidson, E. (1961). *Patients Views of Medical Practice.* New York: Russell Sage Foundation, p. 175.

14. Koos, E. L. (1954). *The Health of Regionville.* New York: Columbia University Press.

15. Davis, M. S. (1968). "Variations in Patients' Compliance with Doctors' Advice," *American Journal of Public Health, 58,* No. 2, 274.

16. Kincey, J. *et al* (1975). "Patients' Satisfaction and Reported Advice in General Practice," *Journal of the Royal College of General Practitioners, 25,* 558.

17. Drury, V. W. M. *et al.* (1976). "Following Advice in General Practice," *Journal of the Royal College of General Practitioners, 26,* 712.

18. Ley, P. *et al.* (1976). "Improving doctor–patient communication in General Practice," *Journal of the Royal College of General Practitioners, 26,* 720.

19. Mechanic, D. (1962). "The Concept of Illness Behaviour," *Journal of Chronic Diseases, 15,* 189.

20. Weber, M. (1969). "Social Action and Social Interaction," In *Sociological Theory,* Eds. Coser, L. A. and Rosenberg, B. London: Collier-Macmillan.

21. Zoborowski, M. (1951). "Cultural Components in Response to Pain," *Journal of Social Issues, 8,* 16.

22. Zola, I. K. (1966). "Culture and Symptoms: an analysis of patients presenting complaints," *American Sociological Review, 31,* 615.

23. Zola, I. K. (1963). "Problems of Communication, Diagnosis and Patient Care: the Interplay of Patient, Physician and Clinic Organisation," *Journal of Medical Education, 38,* 829.

24. Stimson, G. and Webb, B. (1975). *Going to See the Doctor.* London: Routledge and Kegan Paul.

25. McCormick, J. S. (1977). *Journal of the Royal College of General Practitioners,* 27, 318.

26. Cartwright, A. (1967). *Patients and their Doctors.* London: Routledge and Kegan Paul.

CHAPTER II
THE STUDY

The data upon which this account is based have been drawn from a two year study which took place between October 1975 and September 1977. The object of the study was to examine aspects of the doctor/patient relationship from the patients' perspective. There were three principal aims:

(1) To determine effective methods of collecting data by which to assess aspects of interaction between general practitioner and patient, and to assess the practical problems connected with carrying out such a study.

(2) To examine patients' self-perceived expectations of their general practitioner in connection with a particular consultation, and to compare these expectations with their fulfilment and with the doctors' perception of their patients' expectations.

(3) To explore aspects of the explicit and implicit contract between doctor and patient and in so doing enquire into the attitudes of patients towards facets of practice organization.

Two general practitioners from separate practices and their National Health Service patients co-operated in the study. The practices are located in highly urbanized areas of Greater Manchester. The practices and the general practitioners are referred to throughout as "X" and "Y".

The practices

Dr. X's practice is part of a university teaching group-practice of 11 doctors, including three trainee general practitioners. Other medical personnel consist of a full-time social worker, three health visitors, two district nurses, two midwives, a part-time physiotherapist and a part-time radiographer. At the time of the study the practice included approximately 12,000 patients, about 1,900 of whom were registered with Dr. X. The age/sex distribution of the patients over the age of 16 is shown in Table 1.

Table 1
Practice X. Age/sex distribution of patients over 16 years of age

sex	age 16–24		age 25–44		age 45–64		age 65+		totals	
	n	%	n	%	n	%	n	%	n	%
male	274	39	214	31	158	23	52	7	698	100
female	398	50	159	20	146	18	85	11	788	100
totals	672	45	373	25	304	20	137	9	1486	100

Dr. Y practises in a group of four doctors, including a trainee and one general practitioner who is semi-retired. Attached to the group are a midwife, health visitor, district nurse and liaison social worker. Approximately 4,000 patients were registered with the group, 2,800 of whom were registered with Dr. Y. Table 2 shows the age/sex distribution of patients over the age of 16.

20

Table 2
Practice Y. Age/sex distribution of patients over 16 years of age

sex	age								totals	
	16–24		25–44		45–64		65+			
	n	%	n	%	n	%	n	%	n	%
male	154	25	247	39	165	26	62	10	628	100
female	147	20	267	38	189	27	109	15	712	100
totals	301	23	514	38	354	26	171	13	1340	100

The main difference in the age/sex composition of the two practices is in age group 16–24, (p < 0.001). In Practice X this group has both more patients and a higher proportion of females. This difference is due to the location of Practice X near to a complex of university student accommodation and because Dr. X provided medical care to two university hostels for women. However, any effect that these factors may have had on the proportion of patients in each age group who were interviewed was considerably reduced as most interviews took place during the university summer vacation.

The two general practitioners involved in the study were self-selected and their keen interest in research may not be characteristic of general practitioners. The location of Dr. X's practice within a university department of general practice is obviously atypical. In addition, Dr. X directed the research and this may be considered as introducing a further element of bias in at least two respects. Firstly, the questionnaires were assembled by the two researchers and final schedules had been given to both general practitioners. However, by definition, the Director was more fully aware of the content. Secondly, in a study of such an intimate nature it is essential that researchers should be, and be seen to be, entirely neutral observers, whose task is not to arbitrate but to illuminate social action in a particular area. In this climate repondents' views are more likely to be expressed without inhibition and with trust in confidentiality. It is equally important that favourable and unfavourable views are received by the researchers with like response. In order to elicit maximum information the structure of the questionnaires allowed respondents an opportunity to express their views freely. Although confidentiality between the respondents and the researchers was strictly maintained throughout, conflict was undoubtedly and unavoidably created for the latter on the occasions when respondents expressed criticism of Dr. X during interviews. We are not able to judge with any accuracy what effect these factors may have had on the interviews and the relevant consultations. However, there was no evidence that Dr. X's involvement as Director of the study affected doctor/patient interaction in any way.

The patients who were interviewed

A sample of three hundred and twenty patients over the age of 16 were interviewed (Table 3), most of whom were in Social Class III (Table 4).[1] All were registered with either Dr. X or Dr. Y, except 15 who were seen by them because their usual doctor was on holiday.

21

Table 3
Age/sex distribution of patients interviewed and total practice population over 16 years of age

	male				female			
	interviewed		practice pop.		interviewed		practice pop.	
age	n	%	n	%	n	%	n	%
16–24	31	7.2	428	32	45	8.3	545	36
25–44	37	8.0	461	35	54	12.7	426	29
45–64	54	16.7	323	24	56	16.7	335	22
65+	18	15.8	114	9	25	12.9	194	13
totals	140	10.6	1326	100	180	12.0	1500	100

Table 4
Social Class of patients interviewed

Social Class	n	%
I	7	2.2
II	41	12.8
III	136	42.5
IV	63	19.7
V	23	7.2
student	30	9.4
unemployed	19	5.9
unclassified	1	0.3
totals	320	100.0

The study was not designed to compare the two practices involved and no attempt was made to "match" the patients from each practice. For example, Table 5 shows that a larger poportion of patients in Practice X had been registered for three years or less. Although Dr. Y had been with his present practice for 20 years, compared with only eight years for Dr. X, the difference is mainly attributable to the larger number of students registered with Dr. X.

Table 5
Duration of registration

	years registered								totals	
	<1		1–3		4–6		6+			
	n	%	n	%	n	%	n	%	n	%
Practice X	13	52	19	68	13	50	101	45	146	48
Practice Y	12	48	9	32	13	50	125	55	159	52
totals (100%)	25		28		26		226		305	

During interviews with patients three schedules of semi-structured questionnaires were used, (Appendices 1, 3 and 5). These were based on themes which emerged during many hours of informal, exploratory discussion with colleagues, family and friends; few people have not experienced the role of

22

patient at some time. The questionnaires were tested in pilot studies and modified in the light of experience.

Throughout the main study the research design remained constant. Not all questions were appropriate to all respondents. For example, large sections of the questionnaire schedules did not apply to patients who wanted to see the doctor about an administrative matter only. During interviews, respondents had the opportunity to expand any point and comment on any additional aspect they felt was relevant to the enquiry. Content analysis of these additional comments has been made and they will be used for illustration. The interviewers also found that being involved in an enquiry of this nature attracted many "outside" enquiries and anecdotes. Where relevant these are used for occasional illustration.

A total of 480 interviews were carried out between June and November, 1976. The personal characteristics of interviewers, their opinions and expectations of responses as possible sources of bias have been considered in many studies.[2,3] As there were only two interviewers it was possible for each to be accompanied by the other in turn as observer during the pilot studies. From subsequent discussion an endeavour was made to attain a high degree of standardization in the way questions were asked and in the general approach towards respondents. In large scale studies involving many interviewers such close collaboration is obviously impractical and the use of closely structured questionnaires which minimize interviewer bias is therefore more appropriate.

Although only two general practitioners were concerned in this study, the attitudes of 320 people towards their general practitioner are documented. Nevertheless, their views will undoubtedly be affected by their doctors' personality. Bearing these factors in mind, it is accepted unreservedly that generalizations cannot be made from the findings of the study beyond the doctor/patient relationships of the two practices. However, this should not preclude consideration of pointers for further study which are indicated by the findings.

The way in which patients are received at the practice by, or on behalf of the doctor, may influence their attitude towards the practitioner and may even determine whether a particular medical problem is presented, or an expectation expressed. This aspect of general practice management is discussed in Chapter IV, together with the significance of the role of the receptionist as agent of the doctor. The emergent thesis that patients may not value the more personal aspects of the doctor/patient relationship as much as has been assumed by the profession is explored in Chapter V. Chapter VI follows with an assessment of patients' expectations of a specific consultation. This is related both to the doctors' perception of their patients' wants and whether these were met by the doctor during that consultation. An attempt is made to show how patients' expectations may be altered during the consultation and to relate fulfilment of wants to satisfaction.

The quality of communication between doctor and patient clearly plays a major part in whether expectations will be mentioned at all. Factors which may inhibit the expression of patients' expectations are identified. In conclusion, the main points arising from the study are discussed briefly and recommendations are made regarding areas for further study.

"Care of the doctor/patient relation has for too long been left to chance; because of its importance to general practice it must now be examined, defined, and taught, for only then can it be practised efficiently."[4]

REFERENCES

1. General Register Office (1970). Classification of Occupations.

2. See discussion of the 'sympathy effect' in Yule G. V. and Kendall M. G. (1950). *An introduction to the theory of statistics.* London: Griffin.

3. Hyman H. H. *et al* (1954). *Interviewing in social research.* Chicago: University of Chicago Press.

4. Editorial Comment (1967). "Patient demand," *Lancet i*, 483.

CHAPTER III
METHODOLOGY

The sample of patients to be interviewed was drawn in two phases, Group A and Group B.

Group A

Group A consisted of patients who were about to consult one of the two general practitioners concerned in the study. Eighty patients were interviewed at each practice, both immediately before the consultation and later in their own homes. It was decided not to interview patients who were consulting on behalf of another, as the numbers included would be small and would not contribute significantly to the study.

During interview sessions at the practices the researchers attempted to establish for patients a neutral and independent position, by keeping as much as possible to the patients' territory (the waiting room and patients' side of the reception desk) and by wearing casual clothing.

Non-identification with practice staff was easier to maintain at Practice X where space was available for interviewing in a reasonably private area off a corridor but within view of passers by. In Practice Y, interviewing took place in a consulting room that was free at the time, and certainly for one patient this caused confusion. After having been interviewed, Miss B left the practice thinking that she had seen the doctor. She returned later, somewhat embarrassed, to explain to the receptionist. Apparently unable to sustain further loss of face, she wrote to the researchers to say that she had decided not to take part in the study.

To ensure that interviewer bias in the selection of respondents was avoided, patients were selected by random method from the list of appointments which had been made by the receptionist prior to each consulting session. During each session an average of four patients were interviewed, and all sessions were covered alternately by the two interviewers. In order to maintain the flow of patients to the doctor it was agreed that the first two and the last patient of the session would be avoided. However, we appreciate that this may be a possible source of bias.

One of the two interviewers approached the pre-selected patients after they had checked in at the reception desk. Each patient was given a brief outline of the purpose of the enquiry and asked if they would take part in the study, on the understanding that strict confidentiality would be maintained.

Only 13 patients in Group A refused to take part: six gave no reason for their decisions, four could not spare the time, one did not wish to take part because of a personal connection with the practice, one felt too ill to do so and another preferred not to take part in the study because she was consulting about the contraceptive pill unknown to her mother who was waiting for her and might intervene. These patients were excluded from the study and others substituted.

Confidentiality raised ethical problems in two cases. One patient intended to consult her doctor about the birth control pill and a lump in her breast; the other about a vulval cyst with which she had been increasingly troubled over the past year. Although very worried that this might be malignant, embarrassment had prevented her from consulting previously. In the

25

post-consultation interview it was discovered that they had not discussed these potentially serious conditions with their doctor. In both cases they were not able to overcome their embarrassment sufficiently to talk about the problem. In neither case would the patient allow the interviewer to discuss the matter with the doctor concerned and the most that could be done was to impress upon the respondent the need for prompt professional advice.

During the sessions at which interviews took place all consultations between the doctor and patient were, with the patients' permission, recorded on audio-tape. Transcripts from the tapes were made only of consultations relevant to the study, the remainder were erased.

The first interview was carried out at the practice concerned before the patient went in to see the doctor. The questionnaire schedule (Appendix 1) was designed to elicit patients' views of receptionists and the appointments system, which was used at both practices. It also covered patients' general attitudes towards "personal doctoring" and their relationship with their own doctor. The rest of the questionnaire related to the patients' reason for attending, their perception of the seriousness of the condition about which they were going to consult, both medically and socially, and their expectations of the consultation. This interview was kept fairly brief, about seven minutes, as we were aware that patients might be anxious about missing their turn or keeping the doctor waiting.

Each patient was assured that the doctor knew interviews were taking place and that this was bound to affect the timing of appointments to some extent. Also, it was made clear that if as a result of being interviewed respondents missed their turn, the interviewer would ensure that they were the next to be seen. Despite these assurances, however, many patients were concerned about these two aspects and were not entirely relaxed during this first contact.

On completing the pre-consultation interview, an appointment was made to see the respondent at his/her home within the next two days. A letter explaining more fully the aims of the study and indicating the date and time of the next interview was handed to the respondent (Appendix 2).

To eliminate as much as possible any doctor bias in the consultation, the general practitioner was not told which patients were being interviewed, although he knew that an interviewer was present on the premises. Respondents were asked by the interviewer not to mention to the doctor that they had been interviewed. It was hoped that this measure would reinforce both the interviewer's neutral position and assurances of confidentiality. In fact, only 13 of the 160 patients who were interviewed mentioned this to the doctor during the following consultation. In most cases it was just referred to in passing, but two patients wanted to make the point that their co-operation with the interviewer did not imply criticism of the doctor and two mentioned the interview by way of apology for keeping the doctor waiting. Both doctors reported that in subsequent contacts with patients there was very little feedback about the enquiry. On the few occasions that this was referred to, patients were apprehensive about the effect on their relationship with the doctor. Kaim-Caudle and Marsh[1] point out the danger a survey of this nature may have in affecting the relationship of confidence and trust between doctor and patient. With this in mind care was taken throughout the study in both the phrasing of questions and the manner of asking them.

26

The post-consultation interview took place at the patient's home within 48 hours of the consultation to which it related and lasted about 20 minutes. The questionnaire (Appendix 3) brought out more fully aspects which had been introduced in the preconsultation interview. In addition, hypothetical questions were asked about the extent of information and explanation which respondents would like to receive about their conditions and treatments, and the likelihood, based on their past experience, that this would be matched by the doctor in reality. Questions were also asked to elicit the extent of untreated or self-treated conditions. The remainder of the questionnaire specifically concerned the condition or problem which was the subject of the consultation and the outcome in relation to expectations which had been expressed in the first interview. As all consulting respondents were interviewed both before and after the consultation, the relationship between prior expectations and their fulfilment can be followed for the entire group.

Although the second interview was longer than the first, this did not appear to be detrimental. It was found that respondents were far more relaxed on their own home territory. The interview often extended to an hour with little or no prompting from the interviewer and, for many, appeared to be quite a social occasion. One respondent, a Polish lady, said that she was honoured to have been chosen and had generously baked a superb Polish afternoon tea especially for the occasion.

In the more relaxed atmosphere and privacy of their own homes, people seemed more than ready to talk about their illnesses and social circumstances. This was most evident in the two cases where respondents were willing to answer all the questions in the pre-consultation interview except those relating specifically to their main reason for consulting the doctor. Without being pressed in any way, both respondents offered this information during the second interview and seemed to want to discuss the condition and its social implications far more fully than the questionnaire required.

In one case the respondent had a joint appointment with the doctor and a visiting psychiatrist on the day she was interviewed for the study. When asked in the pre-consultation interview why she had come to see the doctor, she said that she had an appointment with the specialist about her general health. She was obviously uneasy about this statement but the interview was not put in jeopardy by pressing for more information on this point. The second respondent had that morning been discharged from a psychiatric unit and had come to the doctor to collect a prescription and sick note. Both conveyed the sense of shame and stigmatized or "spoiled identity" that they perceived to be attached to their condition and which has been so eloquently described by Goffman.[2] A section of transcript from the relevant consultation in the second case is given below. It shows clearly the patient's conscious or unconscious attempts to avoid a fuller discussion of the condition with the doctor, whom he was seeing for the first time.

Dr. "Hm hm. And what was it you were in hospital about?"
Pt. "Um, well, I don't know what it was. You know, I was just run down through working, er, nights and not being able to sleep days."
Dr. "I see. What was the cause of your being run down do you think?"
Pt. "I don't know. I think I overdid it, you know."

Dr. "Hm hm. What symptoms were you having that took you off to hospital?"
Pt. "Um, I can't remember."
Dr. "Well, did they say what the diagnosis was? What was the matter with you?"
Pt. "No, they didn't um . . ."
Dr. "What do you think was the matter with you?"
Pt. "I went to the hospital to see Mr. Brown and he gave me an introductory letter to the hospital and I was accepted."
Dr. "Hm hm. What do you think was the matter with you?"
Pt. "I've no idea."
Dr. "You've no idea at all. Hm hm. Under which consultant were you when you were in the hospital?"
Pt. "Dr. Smith."
Dr. "Dr. Smith?"
Pt. "Hm hm."
Dr. "I wonder how he spells it, do you know?"
Pt. "Um—S–M–I–T–H."
Dr. "Which ward were you in?"
Pt. "Um . . ."
Dr. "Do you have a hospital out-patient card at all?"
Pt. "Er, yes, somewhere here." (Hands card to doctor)
Dr. "Maybe that will help. Thank you very much. 1643S was your number?" "Ah yes."
Pt. "Er, this is the, er . . ."
Dr. "Ah, that's probably giving me the information I'm looking for, isn't it?"
Pt. "Probably, yes. I'd forgotten all about it. Sorry."

We had expected some reluctance on the part of patients to answer the direct question: "What have you come to see the doctor about today?" As a device, we had inserted a lead-in to this question: "Have you prepared in your mind what you will say to the doctor when you go in to see him?" The theory being that when replying to the first question, patients would consider how they would phrase their problem when presenting it to the doctor. Then, with this already in mind, telling the interviewer the reason for consulting would follow more easily.

So far as we are aware, the two cases mentioned above were the only ones where respondents were unwilling to reveal the nature of their complaint. However, we realize that this factor may have contributed to the total of 13 patients originally selected for Group A who did not wish to take part in the enquiry.

To complete the collection of data for Group A, a consultation record was completed by the general practitioner, (Appendix 4). At the end of each interview session a list of patients who had been interviewed was given to the doctor concerned. The consultation record form was completed for each patient on the same day that the interview took place. The form included information about the practical aspects of the consultation, such as examination procedures, diagnosis and action taken, (e.g. the issue of statements of advice concerning work for National Health Insurance purposes, prescriptions, investigations or hospital referrals arranged etc). The doctor was asked also to record his assessment of the patients' expectations of the consultation and the seriousness of the condition or problem, both medically and socially.

Besides providing practical information on what transpired during the consultation, albeit from the doctor's point of view, the record functioned as a bridge between the pre- and post-consultation interviews in the sense that it enabled direct comparison to be made between patients' expectations of the consultation and their fulfilment and the doctor's perception of these expectations. The form also provided the opportunity to compare patients' and doctors' perceptions of the seriousness of the condition. In practice, the consultation record presented considerable methodological problems and a discussion of these follows later.

Group B

Group B comprised 160 patients over the age of 16. Eighty patients from each practice were selected by random method from the practices' records. These patients were interviewed in their own homes. The interview normally took about 20 minutes but was often extended by respondents to an hour. The questionnaire used for this group included all the questions of a more general nature addressed to Group A but not those relating to a specific consultation, (Appendix 5).

None of the patients in Group B had arranged an appointment to see their doctor. This group was included in the study to redress any bias that may have resulted from confining the study to patients who had arranged such an appointment. By confining the sample to attending patients only, patients who were housebound would be omitted and bias would occur in favour of patients who have a higher attendance rate, that is, women and the elderly. It has been a constant finding of previous surveys that women consult more frequently.[3,4] In their comparative study of the characteristics of regular attenders and of those who seldom or never consult their general practitioner, Kessel and Shepherd[5] found that the non-attender group were preponderantly male. Morrell[6] found that this applied in every age group except 0–5.[i] Most studies also show high consultation rates for the very young and very old. Morrell[6] and Hodgkin[7] found that these groups had both the highest proportion of patients consulting and the highest rate of annual consultations per person.

Stimson and Webb[8] estimated that by restricting their sample to consulting patients, bias was likely to have occurred. They reported that a check by one of the receptionists showed that on average the patients interviewed in their research had seen the doctor 8.2 times in the previous twelve months. Estimates of average annual consultation rates per person in England and Wales vary. From the evidence available, Cartwright[9] estimated it to be about five visits per year. Health care data published by the Office of Health Economics[10] shows that the number of consultations in general practice had fallen by 12% between 1955 and 1971 (166.7 million to 146.9 million), which implies an average annual rate of three consultations per person. Taking an average of four consultations per year, it appears that Stimson and Webb's sample visited the doctor twice as often as the norm. An overall count of annual

(i) In view of these and other supporting findings, the cumbersome use of "his/her" is avoided in the text. Respondents are referred to as female, unless a specific case is discussed.

consultations was not made in our study. However, in theory, bias should have been redressed by the controlled selection of patients in Groups A and B.

Group B patients were contacted initially by letter outlining the aims of the project and asking for their co-operation, (Appendix 6). A form suggesting a specific date and time for the interviewer to call, with alternatives should this not be convenient, was enclosed. The time of interview offered took account of the respondent's age as an indication of whether an evening appointment might be more convenient. A stamped and addressed envelope was enclosed for the return of the form.

When making an initial contact by post indicating an intention to call it is essential that authenticity be established, not only because this may influence the response rate but also to minimize any concern that the receipt of the communication may arouse, for whatever reason. Despite the explanation given in paragraph two of the letter, many respondents asked how they had been selected for the enquiry. A few asked if they had been selected because they had upset the doctor in some way, usually by not attending for some time, or whether it was because they had a particular illness. One elderly lady told the interviewer that she had taken our letter to the local police station for advice before agreeing to be interviewed. Another agreed to co-operate only if her brother remained in the room. At the end of the interview this lady offered the interviewer a Drambuie and said that she had actually enjoyed the interview but had been very worried in case we really wanted to use her as a guinea-pig to try out some new drug.

University headed notepaper with telephone and extension numbers was used to allay concern and establish the genuineness of the enquiry but we have no means of knowing how this influenced the response rate. Enclosing a stamped, addressed envelope for reply seemed a natural courtesy and a commonsense step to increase response rate. It is likely that respondents viewed the stamp as representing money and therefore not to be thrown away or used "dishonestly" for some other purpose.

As had been expected from a pilot survey, the initial response rate for Group B was low, (39%). Non-responders were followed up with a telephone call to confirm the arrangement or by the interviewer calling at the respondent's home at least twice. By this method the response rate was almost doubled to 70%. Surprisingly, it was found that calling on respondents at the time given on the form accompanying the introductory letter was most likely to be successful. Respondents appeared to half expect the visit and had the stamped envelope ready to hand over with an apology for not replying.

Nineteen (12%) respondents refused to participate, of whom ten returned the form saying that they did not wish to take part, and nine refused to be interviewed when the interviewer called. We were unable to contact a further 29 (18%) patients. Both practice areas had been involved in demolition and re-housing programmes and the doctors' records had not always kept up with the movement of patients. There also appeared to be a small floating population of itinerant fair-stall holders and travellers who use the address given on the doctor's record only for the collection of mail. Table 6 shows the response rate of the initially selected patients in Group B. Substitutes were drawn by the same random method to bring the number of successful interviews to 80 for each practice.

30

Table 6
Group B response to initial postal enquiry and follow up

	Interviewed (70%)		Refused (12%)		No Contact Made (18%)		
	appoint-ment	follow up	by post	follow up	returned by P.O.	follow up: moved	follow up: away
Practice X (80)	40	13	7	4	5	9	2
Practice Y (80)	23	36	3	5	2	10	1
totals (160)	63	49	10	9	7	19	3

Some bias is inevitable in any postal enquiry. It is most often the less educated, those in lower social categories, and those who are not interested in the subject of the enquiry who are less likely to respond. Furthermore, in a study of this nature respondents' attitudes towards their general practitioner probably have an effect upon response. The problem of bias can most effectively be reduced by making reasonable but determined efforts to mini-mize non-response in the first instance.

Problems in Methodology

The problem of whether it is more satisfactory from a methodological point of view to ask patients about their expectations of the consultation pro-spectively or retrospectively is not easy to resolve. We were aware that by asking questions about specific expectations prior to the consultation we might influence what transpired. Firstly, by unintentionally prompting the patient and secondly, by clarifying and reinforcing their thoughts before they saw the doctor. Stimson and Webb[8,p.13] give an example of this effect in action.

"One woman was asked what she was going to say to the doctor and was then presented with a probing checklist of other things she might say. Asked if she might ask the doctor to examine her she said, 'Now you mention it, I might ask him that', and indeed she did."

Cartwright[11] points out that the interview may act not only as a rehearsal for the coming consultation but as the performance itself. One respondent had said during the pre-consultation interview that she intended to talk to the doctor about spots before her eyes but during the post-consultation interview it became apparent that she had not mentioned this. When asked why, she said that she must have forgotten but was confused about this as she knew she had discussed the condition with someone. As has been shown on page 25 above one respondent in our study became even more involved with the interview as a performance by actually leaving the surgery after being interviewed. Cart-wright's example and our rather extreme case show that the outcome may be significantly affected by a pre-consultation interview in which prior expec-tations are discussed.

To avoid this effect respondents may be asked to give their expectations retrospectively. However, this presents another problem in that expectations given retrospectively may not accurately reflect prior expectations. We tested this out in the pilot survey by asking in the pre-consultation interview: "Do you expect to be given a prescription on this occasion?" and in the post-consultation interview: "Did you expect to be given a prescription when you saw the doctor on . . . ?" It was found that in a significant number of cases patients who had expected a prescription prior to the consultation but were not given this by their doctor, changed their minds when interviewed later and said that they had not expected to be given a prescription. We may presume that cognitive dissonance had been at work in the interim. Or it may be that the expectation was just not very firmly established in the patient's mind prior to the consultation and the previous answer to the question was merely forgotten. Whatever the reason for this confusion, these cases showed that we would not have a reasonably accurate account of specific expectations unless we asked about these *prior* to the consultation.

Another problem which emerged was the necessity to have some objective account of what actually transpired in the consultation to compare with patients' interpretation of what had taken place. For this purpose we designed a record form to be completed by the doctor, (Appendix 4). However, in practice during the pilot study it was found that the patient's and the doctor's accounts were occasionally quite discrepant. To give an extreme example, one patient said he had been referred to a physiotherapist, whereas the doctor had recorded referral to a psychiatrist. When we asked the respondent whether he had expected to be referred to a physiotherapist, he said "No, I thought he would send me to a psychiatrist." Whilst it may be interesting, this degree of inconsistency is also rather confusing. In such cases clarification could easily be obtained from the doctor's record. However, in less extreme cases this may not be possible as the information might not have been considered sufficiently important to include on the patient's notes.

By discussing the consultation with the doctor concerned, many discrepancies might be accounted for in retrospect. However, this would be unsatisfactory in at least three respects: we would be relying on the doctor's memory of an event which had taken place two or three days previously; a post-consultation discussion with the doctor might weight the subjective view of the consultation in favour of the doctor; and perhaps most importantly, it might be difficult to adhere strictly to our promise of confidentiality once discussion with the doctor of a particular case was under way.

We therefore arranged for consultations to be recorded on audio-tape. Patients' permission was sought by the doctor, who explained that the recordings were being done for research purposes. Strangely, patients gave the interviewers no indication that they connected this with the project. As the doctor did not know which patients we were interviewing, the tape recorder was kept running for the whole consultation session and transcripts were made only of the consultations relevant to the enquiry.

So far as the patients were concerned, recording of the consultations appeared to have no effect, and none refused. As for the doctors, both have been in general practice for over eight years and have such well-established patterns of behaviour that they are unlikely to be affected by the presence of a tape recorder. One doctor told the interviewers that apart from one or two initial consultations when he was concerned with technicalities, such as where to place the tape recorder and setting the volume control, he became oblivious to its presence. The other doctor said he was quite unaware of the machine from the start. Neither doctor felt that his behaviour had been modified in any way during the period when interviews took place.

So far as we could judge from the recordings, the interaction displayed no indications of self-conscious or inhibited behaviour on either side. In their study of the verbal behaviour of general practitioners, Byrne and Long[12] found no evidence of inhibited or stilted communication in 2,500 recordings of doctor/patient interviews. Many recordings conveyed evidence to the contrary, in that they amounted to clear examples of "doctor failure" which appeared to be in no way "edited" by the general practitioner concerned. Recordings were also used by Korsch and Negrete[13] in their investigation of the problem of communication between doctors and mothers of children in hospital. Eight hundred interviews were studied and use of the tape recorder was omitted in a control group of 300 in order to assess its effect. There was apparently no difference in doctors' performance or patients' reactions in the two groups. In our study there was further evidence that the doctors were unaware of the tape recorder in that on several occasions they failed to realize that the tape had run out. The set of transcripts is therefore not complete.

In one of the surgeries, clinical examination took place in an examination room adjoining the consulting room and the microphone was not sensitive enough to pick up all the verbal exchanges. For studies which utilize the verbal interaction fully as an integral aspect, these technical difficulties could easily be overcome at the outset. As complete transcripts were made of only two-thirds of the relevant consultations, an empirical examination of the exchanges using, for example, Bales'[14] method of analysis would be unsatisfactory. The transcripts are used mainly for illustration. They also provide a truly objective picture of the consultation and therefore an accurate check on the patient's interpretation of what transpired and the doctor's consultation record form.

A methodological problem which we were not able to overcome entirely satisfactorily related to inconsistency between the pre-consultation interview, the consultation record and the post-consultation interview when more than one complaint was presented to the doctor. The pilot study showed that patients rarely presented more than three conditions. We therefore provided for this maximum contingency by allowing for information relating to primary, secondary and tertiary conditions in the questionnaires and consultation record form. The order of conditions given by the respondent initially in the pre-consultation interview was to be maintained throughout. During the pilot study no problems of inconsistency between the schedules emerged. In the main study, information relating to the primary condition corresponded in both pre- and post-consultation interviews and the consultation record. However, analysis of information relating to secondary and tertiary conditions showed many inconsistencies between the schedules and record form. In effect, when assessing, for example, the seriousness of a secondary or tertiary condition, doctor and patient were not always referring to the same complaint. This mismatch occurred in 42 of the 68 secondary conditions and 5 of the 9 tertiary

33

conditions. We are, therefore, restricted to use of data relating to the primary condition only for purposes of comparison.

Analysis showed that the main reason for the discrepancies was incomplete information given on the doctors' consultation record. Conditions referred to by the patient were not always given in the consultation record, although the transcripts showed that they were in fact discussed during the consultation. To use a typical example, one patient had given ringworm and bronchitis as primary and secondary conditions and the transcript showed that these problems were indeed discussed in the consultation. The patient was actually examined for bronchitis, but only the skin condition was given in the consultation record. In four other cases where respondents said that they had talked to the doctor about a condition which was not given in the consultation record, we checked the transcripts and found that the problem had not actually arisen during the consultation. These inconsistencies may have been due to the rehearsal/performance factor discussed on page 31 above.

A significant number of discrepancies between the schedules also occurred when the patient gave a primary condition only, but which was given as a primary and related secondary condition by the doctor. For example, the menopause was given by both patient and doctor as the primary reason for consulting but with the addition of anxiety state as secondary on the consultation record form. This last kind of mismatch between patients' and doctors' perception of the problem would seem to be inevitable. The additional related condition most commonly appearing on the consultation record was anxiety state. There was also a small number of cases where the doctor's diagnosis given on the consultation record had been withheld from the patient and therefore did not appear in either questionnaire. We were not able to resolve some of the inconsistencies between the schedules as transcripts were not available.

In attempting to resolve this methodological problem for future similar research, we start from the premise that the initial orientation is based on the patient's perspective. Therefore, pre-consultation information given by the patient regarding primary, secondary and tertiary conditions forms the foundation for the additional information given by the doctor. After the consultation, when providing the doctor with the list of patients who have been interviewed for the study, it would be a simple matter to give also the condition(s) as perceived by the patient. In their separate assessments of, for example, the seriousness of the condition(s) we would then be sure that doctor and patient were referring to the same thing, although perhaps using different labels. This method would also overcome to a great extent the doctor's failure to give the required information about a condition on the consultation record, for whatever reason. Additional conditions then given by the doctor only could be analyzed separately. Patients' perception of the condition may, of course, be altered during the consultation and this would emerge during the post-consultation interview.

Problems of a more general nature relate mainly to the construction of questionnaires and formulation of questions. As the questionnaires were administered directly by the interviewers, a fairly complex structure was utilized. This catered for the self-coding of responses, which considerably facilitated the task of transferring information on to computer cards. The

34

structure also allowed for skipping sets of questions where these were not relevant to particular groups. In this connection it is essential that the questions should flow in logical sequence. As the pilot studies showed that we were dealing mainly with Social Groups III and IV, phrasing of questions was kept simple and informal. The most complex question in the schedules is probably Question 7 in the post-consultation interview:

> "If you wanted to see a specialist and the present system was changed so that you could choose between going to him directly, or going through your doctor as we have to now, which would you prefer to do?"

Despite this complexity, only 11 of our 320 respondents gave a don't know response. Hypothetical questions of this complexity present some difficulty as ability to assess in abstract terms is directly related to the level of cognitive development. Thirty-nine (12%) of our 320 respondents gave replies to this question which indicated that they could not imagine or assess the situation as being any different from the status quo. Typical responses to the question were, "I'd rather go through my doctor. It's always been like that," and "Well, you have to go through your doctor, don't you?"

Responses to hypothetical questions as a prediction of future behaviour should be regarded as an imperfect guide. This was well illustrated by La Piere's study[15] of the relationship between expressed attitudes and related behaviour. During a time when feeling against the Chinese was high in the United States he was in a position to note the reception given to Chinese travellers by hoteliers. In only one of the 250 hotels concerned were the travellers refused service. Yet over 90% of those same hoteliers who responded to a postal enquiry asking if they would give service to Chinese, indicated that they would not. Actions were clearly not the same as commitment to behaviour as given in response to the hypothetical question. The manifestation of an attitude depends not only upon the intensity of the attitude but on situational pressures. Response to a hypothetical question may involve nothing more than symbolic rejection or approval of the presented situation. It may also be an indicator of the ideal, rather than the reality. Whilst interpretation of such results should therefore be treated with some caution, they are certainly not without value. Responses will be based on the individual's personal construct of the phenomena in question and, as such, are an indication of his collective past experience of this. Consistency of responses to hypothetical questions between different studies may also give a general pointer to a fruitful line of enquiry. The hypothetical and situational questions of the present project contribute to the findings of other studies which explore patients' attitudes and expectations of their general practitioner and their perception of his role.

REFERENCES

1. Kaim-Caudle, P. R. and Marsh, G. N. (1975). "Patient Satisfaction Survey in General Practice," *British Medical Journal*, 262.

2. Goffman, E. (1968). *Asylums*. Harmondsworth: Penguin.

3. Logan, W. P. D. and Cushion, A. A. (1958). "Morbidity Statistics from General Practice," Vol. 1 (General). *General Register Office Studies on Medical and Population Subjects*, No. 14 London: H.M.S.O.

4. H.M.S.O. (1974). "Office of Population Censuses and Surveys: Morbidity Statistics from General Practice," *Studies on Medical and Population Subjects*, No. 26, London.

5. Kessel, N. and Shepherd, M. (1965). "The Health and Attitudes of People Who Seldom Consult a Doctor," *Medical Care*, *3*, 6.

6. Morrell, D. C., Gage, H. G. and Robinson, N. R. (1970). "Patterns of Demand in General Practice," *Journal of the Royal College of General Practitioners*, *19*, 331.

7. Hodgkin, K. (1973). *Toward Earlier Diagnosis*. London: Churchill Livingstone.

8. Stimson, G. and Webb, B. (1975). *Going to See the Doctor*. London: Routledge and Kegan Paul.

9. Cartwright, A. (1967). *Patients and their Doctors*. London: Routledge and Kegan Paul.

10. Office of Health Economics (March 1976). "Selected Health Service Activities, 1960–1961 to 1973–1974," *Information Sheet* No. 28.

11. Cartwright, A. (1976). "Some Methodological Problems in Studying Consultations in General Practice," *Journal of the Royal College of General Practitioners*, *26*, 894.

12. Byrne, P. S. and Long, B. E. L. (1976). *Doctors Talking to Patients*. London: H.M.S.O. p. 9.

13. Korsch, B. M. and Negrete, V. F. (1972). "Doctor-Patient Communication," *Scientific American*, *227*, 66.

14. Bales, R. F. (1950). *Interaction process analysis*. Boston: Addison-Wesley.

15. La Piere, R. T. (1934). "Attitudes *v.* Actions." *Social Forces*, *13*, 230.

CHAPTER IV
RECEPTION OF PATIENTS

Patients generally have a preconceived idea of the role of the doctor. The patient's view point is derived from an amalgam of impressions gleaned from such sources as the media, family, friends and work associates. In addition, a patient's own direct experience of a relationship with a doctor will contribute towards their construct of the role. The doctor's presentation of his role begins with the way he structures the area in which he works and the management of patients in the process leading up to consultation. Patients receive distinct clues which set the tone of the relationship by defining the situation well before consultation begins. From these combined impressions patients construct their own idea of the relationship and the nature of the service which doctors provide. These impressions may or may not match the patient's ideal or even the reality.

This chapter first examines the system of receiving patients at the two practices in the study. The implication of the system and its influence on patients' attitudes towards their doctor are explored. The appointments system together with the important, but little documented, role of the receptionist are examined in relation to their effect on patients' actions and perception of the doctor.

The setting for reception of patients

Although the research was not designed as a comparative study, in certain aspects it was found that contrasts between the two practices were so obvious and significant it was undesirable to ignore them. The setting and system for receiving patients was one such area.

On arrival at Practice X patients reported at the reception desk and were checked against the list of patients booked for the session by one of the four or five receptionists on duty. They were then given a coloured, numbered tab and told to wait in the waiting room. The number on the tab indicated the sequence of patients; the colour matched the door of the appropriate doctor's consulting room. The doctor was not required to get up from his chair to usher in the next patient. A push button on his desk was wired to a panel of coloured lights and corresponding doctor's name set in front of the rows of chairs in the waiting room. When the button was pressed a coloured light appeared which matched both the tab and the consulting room door. This provided the stimulus for the patient to proceed. Thus, by remote control, patients were processed from receptionist to doctor. This system was to some extent dictated by the fact that the waiting room and most of the consulting rooms were separated by a fifty-foot corridor.

In contrast to this impersonal system the arrangements at Practice Y were less formal. The receptionist's desk opened on to a small chair-lined waiting area where patients sat after reporting in. When the doctor was ready to see another patient he came out of his consulting room and called the next name from his list of patients for that session. The system at Practice X seemed to work well generally but for new patients it could be a little bewildering, especially if the receptionist did not explain the system clearly. Patients who had poor command of the English language were even more perplexed when the receptionist's instruction was no more enlightening than, "Yellow light, yellow door."

For many patients a consultation with the doctor *per se* can be a cause of anxiety. In the post-consultation interview we asked respondents whether they felt nervous about seeing the doctor. Twenty-five per cent confessed that they did. This apprehension is very likely to be heightened by prolonged anti-cipation of the event and by procedures of remote control. Stimson and Webb[1] point out that even the arrangement of waiting room furniture in straight rows may evoke unpleasant associations. From observation of waiting patients at the two practices it was apparent that those of Practice X generally exhibited signs of apprehension which were markedly less evident at Practice Y. As a 50 year old warehouse manager said:

> "Patients get tensed up waiting. If you could just walk in it would be better but the patients all sit in rows and say 'Is he in a good mood today?'"

It was only patients of Dr. X whose comments indicated feelings of resent-ment which reflected the mechanistic nature of the practice system for receiv-ing patients. Such comments as:

> "The doctor's just like a machine working to time."
> "The doctor just looks at you as if you were a number", and
> "I object very strongly to being a number in a book. You're no longer a person these days."

illustrate the point well. In addition, patients who are processed to the doctor by a mechanical system consciously, or unconsciously, absorb the implications of this in relation to their relative status positions. Management problems aside, it is difficult to imagine the general practitioner responding with such robot-like precision to the remote control signal of his patient.

The transcripts showed clearly that the different systems of remote or personal control directly affected the commencement of the interaction between doctor and patient.

At the beginning of each consultation session Dr. X was supplied with a list of patients for the session together with the records of each patient in the same order. Inevitably patients would be late or not arrive at all, so that this order was unlikely to be adhered to. If he could not identify the patient by sight, Dr. X was obliged at the onset of the consultation to ascertain the patient's name. During the study 61% of his consultations began formally with, "Sit down please. And your name is . . . . ?" and a further 12% with such as "Mr . . . . isn't it?"

On one occasion the matter of establishing identity was not quite so straightforward, and the consultation commenced with a most unsatisfactory start from the point of view of both patient and doctor.

Dr. "Come in, good afternoon."
Pt. "Afternoon."
Dr. "Sit down, please. And your name is . . . . ?"
Pt. "Joan X."
Dr. "And what is it you've come for advice about, John?"
Pt. "Um, well, last week I was feeling rather sick, and, er, not eating anything."

Dr. "Where do you live, John?"
Pt. (gives address)
Dr. (On telephone to receptionist) "Will you bring me the cards of John X of
.... please."
Pt. "It's Joan. Joan X."
Dr. "Joan. Oh, I beg your pardon."
Pt. "Joan."
Dr. "Go on, go on."

One man expressed the opinion that it should be a matter of courtesy for the doctor to acquaint himself with the name of a patient prior to the consultation. He expressed his resentment thus:

"He said 'How are you?' I knew he didn't know me from Adam, so I helped him out. While he looked through the file I told him I'd just come out of hospital and that I needed a sick note. Although he asked how I was, he wasn't really interested. I resented him not knowing who I was and I felt sorry for him: not because of his pressure of work but because he wasn't carrying out what I saw as an important part of his work. If I had 10 of my 2,000 employees coming to see me in an hour, I'd make it my business to know who was coming through the door."

The system at Practice Y was more conducive to a more relaxed introduction. As Doctor Y called patients into the surgery by name in order from the appointments list, formal identification was not necessary and consultations began with a typically friendly: "Mrs. Jones, now then, what can I do for you today?" Although Doctor Y may not have been able to identify patients by sight, this was not obvious. The impression given to patients was that the doctor knew them personally.

It is impossible to assess the extent to which these factors affected the consultation itself. Byrne and Long[2, p.34] contend that nothing is to be gained from studying the way doctors greet their patients. However, from the patients' point of view, the doctor has the initiative in establishing the tone of the consultation and the nature of the relationship. It would seem to be inevitable that the interaction will be affected by these initial non-verbal and verbal cues.

The appointments system

In their report *Trends in General Practice*, the Royal College of General Practitioners[3] estimated that over 70% of general practices are arranged round appointments schedules. Both practices in the present study had been organized on the basis of an appointments system for over seven years. Clearly the role of the receptionist is integral to the operation of this aspect of practice management. So far as actual contact with patients is concerned, the main practical task of the receptionist is to regulate the flow of patients to the doctor by constructing appointments lists for each consultation session, managing the practice's system for receiving patients and arranging visits. Within certain limits, the receptionist therefore acts as gatekeeper and controller of the services of the National Health Service general practitioner. These limits are set mainly by appointment times available and, in some practices, by exercise of a degree of responsibility in assessing needs of patients.

During the time that interviews were being carried out for the study Doctor X allotted eight hours per week for consultations. These were held on three mornings, one afternoon and one evening, with appointments normally every ten minutes but decreasing to five minutes if demand required. Doctor Y held consultations for ten hours per week at three morning and three evening sessions, with appointments every five minutes. The evening surgery at both practices was a misnomer in that the last appointment was made for 5.55 p.m. Consultation hours are obviously set by the doctor in the context of managing the practice as a whole. But from the point of view of patients who work a full day, these evening surgery hours may be very inconvenient and may even result in loss of earnings. The implications are that if patients consider their condition warrants a visit to the doctor, they will be prepared to take time off work in order to see him. However, this is to take an unrealistic and unsympathetic view of the economic work situation of many patients, thereby causing some resentment. One of our respondents who had tried without success to make an appointment for her husband for the end of the evening surgery commented:

> "The receptionist was so unreasonable and said 'Couldn't he take a day off work to come and see the doctor?'"

Cartwright[4, p.105] found that only 4% of a sample of 1,162 respondents said that the latest time they could be seen at the doctor's surgery was 6 o'clock. Fifteen per cent could be seen up to 6.30 p.m. Half expressed disapproval of a 5.30 p.m. finish because of the difficulties for people who worked.

We did not ask respondents specifically whether they preferred an appointments system as there is already much evidence to show that most patients are in favour, especially at practices where the system already operates.[4,5,6] However, of those who volunteered the information that they disliked the appointments system, the majority were in full-time employment. Table 7 shows a highly significant correlation between difficulty in obtaining an appointment and age group. It was respondents in age group 26–45, those most probably in full-time employment, who were most likely to have difficulty in obtaining a convenient appointment. Fifty-five per cent said that they had experienced problems, compared with 14% of those over 65 years of age.

Table 7
"Have you ever wanted to see the doctor before the earliest appointment offered to you?"

Age	No	Yes
16–25	37	30
26–45	40	49
46–64	68	42
65+	36	6
Totals	181	127

$n = 308$
x^2 20.37   3 df $p < .001$

Apart from provision for emergencies which was made at both practices, Practice X was rigid in applying the appointments system, whilst Practice Y

40

took a more flexible approach. In theory, the policy of Practice Y was that if patients were prepared to take the trouble to come to the surgery then they must perceive themselves to be sick. They were, therefore, to be seen by the doctor although all appointments for the session had already been filled. Examination of the appointments lists at Practice Y during the study showed that it was indeed quite normal for 8–15 extra patients to be seen and consultation sessions rarely finished at the due time. On average, the number of consultations per week for Doctor X was 52 and for Doctor Y 150. Yet in spite of their more flexible approach to the appointments system and the greater number of patients seen each week, it was the patients of Doctor Y who found him to be less accessible. Forty-seven per cent had difficulty in making an appointment, compared with 35% of Practice X patients. The difference between the two practices is shown in Table 8.

Table 8
"Have you ever wanted to see the doctor before the earliest appointment offered to you?"

	No	Yes
Practice X	99	53
Practice Y	82	74
Totals	181	127

n = 308
x^2 4.51   1 df   p < .05

Examination of the data available from the study shows that, taking into account the number of patients registered at each practice and estimating an average of four visits per patient per year, Doctor X could expect to see 146 patients per week with three minutes for each consultation. In fact he was seeing just over one-third of this number and was able to allocate an average of nine minutes to each patient. Doctor Y could expect 215 consultations per week, averaging only three minutes each. He actually saw approximately 150 patients, with consultations averaging four minutes each. Byrne and Long[2, p.109] estimate that the average consultation takes $5\frac{1}{2}$ minutes and that diagnosis occurs after an average of three minutes.

An interpretation of the data indicates that the demand for consultations made by Doctor Y's patients does not appear to exceed the norm. However, the rate of return consultations requested by each doctor may have been a contributing factor to their work load. Whilst Doctor X asked 55% of his patients to make a further appointment to consult, Doctor Y asked 69% to see him again. These figures could have occurred by chance in the sample, (p < .20 > .10). Morrell[7] reported that 47% of all consultations are doctor initiated. It appears that Doctor Y greatly exceeds this average. This may be an element of his emotionally supportive style of doctoring. Clearly, in the time he allocates for consultations, Doctor Y is not able to see as many of his patients as would like to consult him and this is inevitably reflected by pressure on the practice system.

41

From the individual patient's perspective, the effects of this pressure are felt first with difficulty in obtaining an appointment and secondly, by observing the constantly crowded surgery and rapid turnover of patients. As one of Doctor Y's patients observed:

"When the appointments first started it was just fine but over the last six months there seems to be a lot of waiting and chaos for Doctor Y's surgeries."

During interviews at Practice Y, surgeries were held by Doctor Y only, occasionally accompanied by a trainee doctor. This was a factor in affecting patients' ability to observe directly the pressure under which Doctor Y worked during consultation sessions. A review of the many related comments from our sample shows that the patients of Doctor Y were far more likely to regard their doctor as being a very busy man. Their part in the consultation may be affected in various ways by this impression. The following typical comments show the general sense of urgency felt by patients as a reflection of the doctor's rapidity in dealing with patients and the weight of patients yet to be seen:

"I always get out as fast as I can. I always get the impression that once you're in you've got to get out fast."

" . . . you feel you're wasting his time. The surgery is always so full and he's always in such a hurry. You feel on pins and wish you hadn't come."

In the last quoted and many other cases, patients at both practices would have liked the doctor to explain some aspect of their condition but felt unable to ask about it because the doctor appeared to be so busy. Some patients used the number of waiting patients as a barometer by which to assess whether or not they would present more than one condition.

Apart from the many comments relating to these direct pressures, we found some evidence at both practices of a tacitly agreed norm amongst patients which regulates the number of conditions to be presented at one consultation, the number of prescriptions requested and the duration of a consultation. Some examples illustrate: a patient said that she had not consulted the doctor about painful piles because: "I've been with so many other things and so often, I'm ashamed to go with anything else"; a 75 year old woman who was being treated for myxoedema, arthritis and myocardial ischaemia had intended to ask for a prescription for sleeping tablets but had failed to do so; "I thought I'd got so many pills and new heart pills, I didn't like asking for anything else"; a 54 year old building superintendent with diabetes would like to have had the condition explained to him thoroughly but felt there was no point in even beginning to discuss it with the doctor as this might take an hour. The thought of asking the doctor in advance for a long session in which to discuss the condition had not occurred to him. However, it is interesting to speculate whether this request would be regarded by a National Health Service general practitioner as deviant.

This informal regulation of the time a patient may reasonably spend with the doctor becomes most apparent in the waiting room. If a patient exceeds the norm, the grumbles of waiting patients are likely to start: "She's taking a long time, isn't she?"

Waiting

Generally, patients appear to be amazingly tolerant about being kept waiting. Despite the fact that few are likely to have experienced the matching of their appointment with the time they actually see the doctor, most patients habitually turn up at the specified time prepared to wait for his attention. It is a reflection of their respective status that this routine is expected and accepted.

Although patients may wait in the waiting room for 10–30 minutes, or even longer, after the time of their appointment, it would seem quite inappropriate for the doctor to apologize. The National Health Service patient would probably be very surprised if he did. Patients appear to be reasonable people generally and those who arrived late were apt to do so in a degree of fluster which suggested a spirited attempt to arrive on time despite some contretemps. Patients who were five minutes late for an appointment were likely to be taken to task by the receptionist and feel constrained to apologize to her. Yet in practical terms, the apology appeared to be quite unnecessary as the flow of patients to the doctor was seldom affected, unless the late comer had an appointment at the beginning or end of the surgery session. The receptionist's admonition may be as much a demonstration of the power attached to her role as it is a desire to maintain order on behalf of the doctor. The patient's apology to the receptionist appears to be a gesture of deference to her role as effective intermediary and a symbolic penance to the doctor.

Being late merited disapproval from both receptionists and other patients. At Practice X the receptionist had direct control over the order in which patients saw the doctor. Even though many patients were already waiting, the penalty was incurred by a late arriver of having to wait whilst patients who had arrived after were given priority. To complain would be to risk loss of face by the receptionist's pronouncement: "Yes, but you were late."

The receptionists

Clearly, from the patients' perspective, the receptionist occupies a strategic position in that she has power to facilitate or obstruct access to the doctor in accordance with her control of the appointments system. Despite the fact that 41% of our sample found some difficulty in obtaining a convenient appointment, and almost half of these often had difficulty, most patients appeared to be able to take an objective view of this as far as the receptionists were concerned. Many complained quite forcibly about having to wait for an appointment but did not generally vent their frustration in criticism of the receptionist. It did not appear to occur to any patient to discuss this problem with their doctor, even when they were presented with the kind of dilemma faced by this respondent:

> "The doctor said to bring my daughter in when her glands were swollen but then we can't get an appointment on the day. Her glands may be O.K. next day when we do have the appointment. We have to cancel it then as he said to bring her in when the glands were up."

This lack of communication is not surprising in view of the role expectations attached to doctor and patient. As one patient said: "It's not up to the patient to tell the doctor what to do." The patients of a National Health Service practice are an amorphous congerie who do not pay directly for their doctor's services. As such, with few exceptions, they have no voice in practice management.

The overwhelming majority of patients, 80%, found that when making an appointment or enquiry the receptionists were either very helpful or quite helpful. There was no significant difference between the two practices in this respect. Neither were age, sex and social group of patients significant factors. This figure corresponds closely with that of Kaim-Caudle and Marsh[6] who found that 96% of their sample thought that the receptionists provided an average or good service. There is little evidence in our study of the popular image of "the dragon at the gate". Considering the consistently large number of patient contacts made by the receptionists in the course of their duties and the emotive nature of illness itself, this finding is obviously to their credit. Eleven per cent of our sample said that the receptionists varied in their willingness to be helpful and only 9% found that they were not at all helpful. The small minority, 12%, who made specific complaints were both voluble and vociferous in doing so. Were it not for the objective data, it would certainly be easy to gain a strong general impression of patients' animosity towards receptionists. Whilst keeping in mind that we are dealing with a fairly small minority, the factors which contribute to the finding bear identification.

In his survey of informal and formal complaints against general practitioners, Klein[8] found that the remarks and manners of receptionists accounted for 14.9% of expressions of dissatisfaction. He concluded that these frequently reflected a general sense of disapprobation which converged upon and was rationalized by a particular incident. Of the 41 specific complaints made against the practice receptionists involved in the present study, the majority referred to their personal manner. Such adjectives as offhand, abrupt, bossy and arrogant were commonly used. Whilst recognizing that this may be largely a function of patients' frustration in obtaining an appointment and the pressure upon busy receptionists of dealing with the limited elasticity of appointments schedules, it is obvious that personality cannot be discounted. Receptionists who are patently unsympathetic in their handling of patients may best be regarded as a management problem which should not be ignored by the doctor. As patients are very unlikely to complain directly to their doctor, the problem may be initially one of detection by him.

Other respondents' criticisms related directly to arranging appointments. In most of these cases the receptionist seemed to be perceived as an independent agent in directing policies of practice management and was considered to be perversely obstructive. These patients obviously resented what they perceived as the receptionist dictating when they should be seen and by whom, as the following comments illustrate:

> "The receptionists aren't very helpful. They say you have to 'phone before 10 o'clock if you want an appointment."

> "When I asked to see Doctor X they said I had to see Doctor K. They're not very helpful."

One respondent who was registered with Doctor X but usually saw another doctor at the practice said that the receptionist would not let her make an appointment with the other doctor: " . . . she said I had to see my own doctor." For whatever the reason, the receptionist had not explained that the preferred doctor was on holiday.

The third most common reason for complaints related indirectly to making appointments. In dealing with any relatively scarce commodity, assessment of priority becomes almost inevitable. Receptionists at both practices were often involved in gathering information about the condition from patients, in order to estimate their need for an appointment or visit. The principal receptionist at Practice Y was trained in first aid as part of a medical receptionists' course and was therefore well versed in the priorities of breathing–blood–bones. Apart from this, none of the receptionists were equipped by training to make anything but a commonsense assessment. From most patients' point of view there would be no reason to suppose that the receptionist was likely to have more commonsense than they, or to stand in a better position to judge the case over the telephone. The receptionist's enquiries were therefore regarded by some patients as an attempt to emulate the doctor in diagnozing and assessing the seriousness of the condition. They considered that in doing so she was exceeding her clerical function and obstructing access to the doctor.

A few of our frustrated respondents who had failed to obtain an early appointment after describing their condition, attempted to see their doctor by asking for a visit instead of the offered appointment for two or three days hence. According to our more aggresive respondents, this ploy usually worked. One rather timid patient had less success:

> "On a Thursday I was quite ill and rang for an appointment. The receptionist said I couldn't see the doctor until Monday, so I asked for a visit. She wouldn't let me have one and said the doctor wouldn't come out, although she didn't ask him."

Klein[8, p.114] quoted evidence that the function of receptionists appeared to be more to keep doctor and patient apart than to bring them together. This view is implied in our respondents' complaints. One woman commented directly that receptionists removed the contact that patients wanted with their doctor and that patients should be able to speak to him on the telephone. Doctor E. Byrne[9] reported that it is the established custom of Danish general practitioners to receive calls personally from patients between the hours of 8 and 9 a.m. from Monday to Friday. Patients are then advised by him whether to call in and pick up a prescription, attend for consultation or arrange for a visit. In his own practice Doctor Byrne has found this system to be most effective in practice management and maintaining patient contact. Both doctors of our study were willing to receive telephone calls from patients at convenient times but in fact Doctor Y very rarely spoke to patients on the telephone. At both practices the receptionist first ascertained the patient's reason for wanting to speak to the doctor, in order to assess whether a consultation at the surgery would be more appropriate. Kaim-Caudle and Marsh[6] found that 30% of their sample objected to having to tell the receptionist why they wanted to see the doctor. Although not specifically expressed by our respondents, this factor may also have contributed to the total number of complaints by our respondents.

The filtering role of the receptionist as front line negotiator between doctor and patient is not unique to general practice. The equivalent can be observed to varying degrees and levels in commerce and industry. This is an aspect of management which is generally understood and accepted, albeit at times with frustration. However, there is of course a difference and the essence of this lies in the uniquely intimate and emotive nature of illness itself. In dealing with such a commodity it would be unreasonable not to expect conflict to arise at all. The scale of complaints against receptionists may depend as much on her personal qualities as it does on the system she is required to operate. It also depends on patients' demands on the system and their tolerance of its imperfections. Whilst many patients rationally accept the need of priority assessment for a limited number of appointments or visits, they may be quite unwilling to accept the aspect of the receptionist's role which requires her to assess that need. A sympathetic and tactful approach will undoubtedly facilitate acceptance. In practical terms, training of receptionists to an appropriate level of medical competence would undoubtedly inspire greater confidence in their decisions and advice. It is likely that greatly increased job satisfaction would also result. Failing this training, the policy of occasional monitoring of receptionists' telephone exchanges with patients, followed by discussion, may help to ensure that limits of competence are not being overstepped.

For patients, the ability to contact their doctor directly and to see him that day if desired is a practical ideal which may be seldom matched in the reality of contemporary general practice. The view that the role of the receptionist is intrusive in the doctor/patient dyad implies that a specially intimate relationship exists between the two, beyond the practical role expectations outlined in Chapter I. The nature of this relationship is now explored in the following chapter.

REFERENCES

1. Stimson, G. and Webb, B. (1975). *Going to See the Doctor.* London: Routledge and Kegan Paul, p. 26.

2. Byrne, P. S. and Long, B. E. L. (1976). *Doctors Talking to Patients.* London: H.M.S.O.

3. Royal College of General Practitioners (1977). *Trends in General Practice.*

4. Cartwright, A. (1967). *Patients and their Doctors.* London: Routledge and Kegan Paul.

5. Harris Poll, (1972). *Doctors and their Patients.*

6. Kaim-Caudle, P. R. and Marsh, G. N. (1975). "Patient Satisfaction Survey in General Practice," *British Medical Journal,* 262.

7. Morrell, D. C., Gage, H. G. and Robinson, N. R. (1970). "Patterns of Demand in General Practice," *Journal of the Royal College of General Practitioners, 19,* 331.

8. Klein, R. (1973). *Complaints against Doctors.* London: Chas. Knight & Co. Ltd.

9. Byrne, Dr. E. (Nov. 1977). *Danish G.P.'s Bring Home the Bacon.* Pulse.

CHAPTER V

PATIENTS' ATTITUDES TOWARDS PERSONAL DOCTORING

In this chapter patients' attitudes towards a "personal doctor" are explored in relation to general practice. The term "personal doctor" implies that a special relationship exists between a general practitioner and his patient. This is easier to describe than to define. At its most basic level, the association is one of continuous care by the same doctor which the patient willingly accepts and actively co-operates in maintaining. The patient invests in that doctor responsibility and authority for care of his general health. The doctor's interest in the patient is apparent and essentially personal, in the Parsonian sense already described in Chapter 1.

Evidence of the orientation of general practitioners with regard to personal doctoring is reviewed briefly. Patients' views are then examined: firstly, with regard to the importance attached to continuous care by one doctor and secondly, the doctor's position as first contact medical adviser is assessed in relation to a nurse in general practice and patients' autonomy in dealing directly with a hospital specialist of their own choice. The presence of a third party in the consultation between doctor and patient inevitably dilutes the intensity of the interaction compared with the privacy of the one-to-one encounter traditionally expected in personal doctoring. This factor is explored with reference to patients' attitudes towards the presence of a medical student in the consultation. A further indicator of patients' attitudes towards personal doctoring is taken by whether patients would consider taking their personal problems to their doctor, even if not strictly medical. Finally, patients' views of two basic approaches to the doctor/patient relationship are examined. These are: (1) person-centred or illness-centred care, and (2) impersonal, business-like or friendly styles of interaction. The two approaches are examined both in relation to patients' preference and their perception of the relationship they have with their doctor.

General practitioners' orientation

The Royal College of General Practitioners defines the general practitioner inter alia as:

" . . . a doctor who provides personal, primary and continuing medical care to individuals and families."[1]

In "Present State and Future Needs of General Practice" they continue to emphasize the importance of the doctor's personal interest in the patient and family.[2] There appears to be very little empirical information from general practitioners themselves to support this theoretical stance. Cartwright[3, p. 154] provides the major empirical evidence in the reported views of 416 general practitioners drawn from a nationwide sample. Seventy-one per cent agreed with the following statement, of whom 43% agreed strongly:

"If general practitioners working in partnerships are to establish satisfactory personal relationships with their patients, it is important that patients should be encouraged to stick to the same doctor."

16% disagreed with the statement, of whom 6% disagreed strongly. Not surprisingly, doctors who managed single-handed practices were more likely to agree strongly than their colleagues who worked with three or more others. The statement, however, begs the question: is establishing satisfactory personal relationships by encouraging patients to stick to the same doctor conducive to the practice of better medical care?

Forty-six per cent of the general practitioners in the above study said that personal contact with patients provided the most enjoyable aspect of their work. Many commented that they valued the friendship and respect of their patients and stressed the satisfaction afforded by knowing their families and background. Bridgestock[4] presented a nationwide sample of general practitoners with the 13 aspects of general practice which had arisen spontaneously as sources of satisfaction or dissatisfaction in Cartwright's study. Relationships with hospital staff and access to hospital diagnostic facilities provided the greatest sources of satisfaction. Patients' respect and friendship were rated as being almost equally important.

Individual views supporting the personal doctor approach have been published in medical journals. For example, Hopkins[5] asserted that continuity of care for the patient and family is synonymous with caring for patients as people. He also implied that the doctor's sense of security is threatened by diffusion of personal responsibility for patients and resulting uncertainty of patients' expectations. Clyne[6] implies that some kind of mystical cerebral union takes place between doctor and patient which creates their special personal relationship and only when this has been accomplished can continuity of personal care be broken and the patient referred for attention by para-medical personnel. However, he acknowledges that such "strong emotional bonds" may not be acceptable to some patients.

> "We all know of patients on whom we have lavished a high degree of personal care and who, apparently ungratefully and incomprehensively, have left us to sign on with another doctor in the district."

Whilst both Clyne[6] and Aylett[7] subscribe to the principle of personal doctoring, they confuse the point by implying that compassion and the ability to assume the other's frame of reference exist only within the framework of personal doctoring.

It is beyond dispute that compassion and empathy are two of the most vital components of a doctor's non-medical armoury. But, if he possesses them at all, these traits will be an integral part of his personality. As such they will be activated in response to appropriate stimuli in all personal contacts. Indeed, empathy and compassion may be felt towards individuals, or even groups of individuals, in the complete absence of direct personal contact. To presume that understanding and personal warmth are by definition accompanied by personal doctoring is as illogical as assuming the corollary, i.e. that they are absent in less continuous and less personal doctor/patient interaction. In the last analysis, personal relationships depend first upon personalities, not on roles. No amount of personal family doctoring will bring about a special relationship if the general practitioner is unable to create a sense of rapport between himself and his patients.

48

There does not appear to be any evidence that standards of care in general practice are better or worse according to the degree of personal doctoring extended to patients. Cartwright[3, p.67] concludes that:

"... the data from this study certainly do not suggest that the advantages of a family doctor are so great that they should necessarily outweigh other considerations of efficiency and specialization."

The foregoing views of doctors may be more indicative of their personal needs rather than the needs of their patients. Few studies have been carried out to determine whether the professional orientation is reciprocated by patients. Several questions which were asked in the present study contribute to an understanding of this issue.

The patients' orientation
Continuity of care: One of the principal features of personal doctoring is continuity of care by one doctor. We assessed how much this mattered to patients by asking how they would feel if they had made an appointment with a particular doctor and found on arrival that the consultation was to be with someone else. For respondents in Group A, who were interviewed for the study prior to consulting the doctor, this question was likely to be more meaningful than it was for Group B, who were interviewed at their own home without reference to a particular consultation. Group A would be inclined to base their response to the question on a projection of their attitude towards the consultation which was about to occur. The question would not therefore be entirely hypothetical, as it was for Group B. In fact, we found that there was very little difference between the responses given by the two groups.

One hundred and eighty-nine (59%) of our respondents said that it would not matter if they saw another doctor. Typical comments were that as far as they were concerned one doctor was as good as another Neither age, sex nor marital status were significant factors in this respect.

Eighty-six (27%) respondents said that they would not like to see another doctor. Forty-five (14%) said that their attitude would depend upon which doctor they were to see and the seriousness of the condition or problem. Most of these patients' remarks related to some aspect of continuity. Comments most often referred to the importance of the doctor who was to be consulted not being a stranger. However, there was no indication that this preference was based on a special relationship. There was some evidence that the very fact of having met the doctor previously, alleviated to some extent the anxiety attached to consulting *per se* and reduced feelings of vulnerability. The following comments aptly illustrate the point:

"I feel quite apprehensive about seeing the doctor today as I haven't seen this one before."

"Once you've made contact you feel more assured next time you see the doctor."

"You can explain yourself better to your own general practitioner because you know how to take him."

49

The second most common reason for patients wishing to see the general practitioner of their choice related to his competence as a doctor. Comments showed that their confidence was not necessarily related to a satisfactory personal relationship between doctor and patient. In fact, in some cases it was quite clear that from the patients' perspective the relationship was not conducive to easy communication and the doctor did not appear to take an interest. However, for these patients his medical competence and the confidence this engendered took priority.

A particular doctor's knowledge of the patient's medical history or problem was also important for some patients. In two cases respondents and doctor were concerned in an ongoing investigation into a sudden death. Neither would see another doctor from preference because of the trauma of having to explain the matter all over again and the effect of the incident on their health. One patient who was being treated for depression associated with alcoholism expressed the opinion that, as far as the latter condition was concerned, continuity of care was very important. He felt that it was essential that doctor and patient should discuss progress together on a continuous basis and that the patient should be confident of the doctor's special understanding of the difficulties associated with alcoholism.

Preference for seeing one doctor appeared more often to be based firmly on rational grounds, rather than on personal considerations. Respondents explained:

"You see another doctor and you get fobbed off because he doesn't know your case and you have to come back again."

"It can often waste your time and the doctor's seeing someone who doesn't know your history, as you often have to come back again about the same thing to your regular doctor."

Ninety-seven (61%) of the respondents in Group A had been consulting the doctor for less than one month about the condition which was their primary reason for consulting during the study. Twenty-one people (13%) had been consulting for between one and six months and 42 (26%) for more than six months. It was the patients who had been consulting for the longest period who were least likely to object to seeing another doctor, $(p < .01)$. Seventy-three per cent of this group said that they would not mind seeing another doctor, compared with 40% of those who had been consulting for one to six months and 62% of those who had been consulting for less than one month. It may well be that patients who have been consulting for a long period generally regard the treatment of their condition as one of relatively stable, routine management which could be carried out by any doctor in possession of the relevant notes. If so, they would be likely to feel less dependent on one doctor than patients whose condition was in the process of being investigated or organized.

Patients who explicitly commented on the value of the more personal aspects of their relationship with their doctor as a reason for preferring continuous care were small in number, only 10 (3%). All respondents in this group expressed their appreciation of the doctor's understanding and his personal interest in themselves and their families.

It would seem then, that for most patients continuity of care from the same doctor was not of overriding importance and few patients appeared to regard

50

their relationship with their doctor in personal terms. However, it is readily appreciated that generalizations cannot be made beyond the doctor/patient relationships of the two practices in this study. There is both supporting and conflicting evidence from other studies. Batty[8] reports that observation of his own group practice of eight doctors caring for 18,000 patients, shows a definite and continuing tendency towards patients' preference for multi-doctor care. This observation was supported by a controlled study of a representative sample of 500 patients taken each year between 1971 and 1976. Table 9 shows the trend quite clearly. The patients at this group practice had "unconstrained liberty of choice among available doctors". It is inevitable that this factor contributed to the findings.

Table 9
The trend towards patients' preference for multi-doctor care

Patients seeing:	1971–73	1974–76
	%	%
One doctor	20	13
Two doctors	24	27
Three or more doctors	56	60

J. Batty, 1977.

McKenna and Wacker[9] report from a study of a comprehensive pre-paid group practice attached to Harvard University. The study was aimed at discovering patients' preferences for seeing one or more doctors. Patients were encouraged to maintain a relationship with one doctor but were not actually restricted to this policy. A "wide selection" of physicians was available and consultations could be made by appointment with a particular doctor, or patients could attend a walk-in clinic which was covered in rotation by a regular panel of doctors. An ongoing doctor/patient relationship, or personal physician, was defined mainly in terms of the percentage of consultations held with the same doctor. If a patient had seen one doctor for at least 40% of consultations, preference for having a personal doctor was recorded. Of the 1,191 individuals in the sample, 48% preferred to see more than one doctor. Of the 457 married couples, only 28% shared the same personal doctor. For 37%, one of the couple preferred to have a personal doctor and the other chose to see more than one doctor. The researchers concluded that the results suggest that patients may not value an ongoing relationship with one physician as much as has been assumed.

However, the evidence is not entirely consistent. Kaim-Caudle and Marsh's study[10] of one doctor's patients in a group practice showed that the overwhelming majority, 80%, preferred to see one doctor. It is not possible to assess with any degree of certainty what factors influenced the patients of this practice to vote almost unanimously for continuous care. Perhaps the most simple explanation lies in the personal qualities of this particular doctor.

On the other hand, studies show that in some respects patients tend to prefer the system to which they are accustomed. It is certainly a possibility that patients' preference for the status quo influenced the findings in each of the above three studies. If the group practice policy of Kaim-Caudle and Marsh's study was to discourage patients from seeing more than one doctor, this may have affected their attitude in favour of personal doctoring. Obviously, not only must other doctors be available, but access to them must be unrestricted so that expressed preference is founded on possible options.

In our study we found that the patients of Dr. X were less likely to be concerned if their appointment was changed to another doctor, (p = <.05). One hundred and five patients (66%) said that this would not matter, compared with 82 (51%) of Dr. Y's patients. In theory, access to available doctors was not restricted at either practice. At Practice X one of seven doctors could be seen by appointment and two at Practice Y. Practice X was organized in a system of three teams, apart from one doctor who worked without a team. Each team consisted of two doctors and a trainee doctor. Patients were able to make an appointment within the team of the doctor with whom they were registered. Whilst not formally restricted to this policy, they were discouraged by doctors and receptionists from any departure. At Practice Y, choice could be freely exercised between the two doctors of the practice.

We found that some patients at both practices were not clear about exercising their option to see a doctor other than the one with whom they were registered. Concern was expressed by respondents about both the "legality" and reaction of the doctor if they were to see someone else in the practice. For example, a woman who quite clearly felt she had a poor relationship with the doctor with whom she was registered was asked why she continued to see him despite this. She replied:

> "I don't really want to be with this doctor, but I'm registered with him and I prefer to see just one doctor."

Another patient in the same position said she had asked one of the other doctors in the group whether she could change her registration to him. She had apparently been told by him that this would not be diplomatic and it would be all right for her to see him without altering her registration. She was not convinced that this was the right thing to do and continued to see the doctor with whom she was registered. The difficulties facing patients who wish to change their doctor by re-registering have been discussed in other studies which show that the option to "vote with the feet" is not as simple as it appears to be.[11,12]

Unless a practice's policy of multi-doctoring is made quite clear to patients from source, there may well be some sense of guilt attached to seeing more than one doctor. The following transcript of one of Dr. Y's consultations illustrates the point, although much of the meaning conveyed in the paralinguistic aspects of the dialogue is lost.

Dr. "So really, all you want is a sick note?"
Pt. "Please, yes."
Dr. "Yes. Well, I really think . . . ." (An awkward silence was broken by the patient's apologetic admission . . .).
Pt. "I came to see Dr. M last week."
Dr. "That's all right, yes. etc."
Pt. "No disrespect to Dr. M, Dr. Y. Don't get me wrong."
Dr. "No."

Pt. "But I said I'll see Dr. Y, you know. etc. I know I should have . . . I should tell Dr. M I've seen you too . . . ."

Dr. "No, no, no, no, no, no."

It is evident from other parts of the transcript that this patient had a warm, personal relationship with Dr. Y which she was afraid of having damaged by seeing another doctor.

Continuity of care and the general practice nurse

Patients' attitudes towards seeing a nurse instead of their doctor for minor conditions is also an indication of their views regarding continuous primary medical care by one doctor. We asked respondents how they would feel about a nurse attending to minor conditions in place of the doctor. The overwhelming majority, 265 (83%), said that they would be satisfied with this arrangement. Few of these had any additional comment to make. Forty-five (14%) said that they would prefer to see the doctor, three of whom said they would not mind being attended to be a nurse providing the doctor saw the condition first. Ten (3%) were not sure. Of those who gave a reason for their preference not to be seen by a nurse, almost all said they had more confidence in the doctor's opinion because he was better qualified. Only one of the sample of 320 referred to the hypothetical nurse in terms of her intercepting in the patient's relationship with the doctor.

This finding is strongly supported by Kaim-Caudle and Marsh's study.[10] Virtually all respondents approved of having treatments such as injections or ears syringed by a nurse and 75% would not have minded having minor complaints treated by a nurse instead of the doctor. Follow-up visits by the nurse to cases which had been seen initially by the doctor were overwhelmingly approved of by the patients.

At the recent conference held by the British Medical Journal, the issue of ancillary workers in general practice was discussed.[13] One group practice of four doctors reported having employed two nurses as patients' first contact for the past eight years. This added dimension had worked with considerable benefit and satisfaction for both doctors and patients. From the patients' point of view the filtering role of the nurse was readily accepted. They were quite prepared to discuss their clinical history with her on the telephone or at the practice and be advised as to the necessity to see the doctor. This favourable acceptance is in marked contrast to the resentment and resistance of patients to the receptionists' filtering role, as already discussed in Chapter IV. The doctors found their work more meaningful and enjoyable. They were able to spend more time with patients and generally saw fewer cases which were of a relatively trivial nature. Cartwright's study[3, p.47] showed that 49% of the general practitioners regarded between 25% and 75% of their consultations as trivial, unnecessary or inappropriate. Sixty-five doctors from a random two-fifths of the original cohort of 422 doctors in this study were later asked for information about the nature of their consultations. Of 2,500 consultations, an average of 38 from each doctor, one-fifth were felt to be trivial, inappropriate or unnecessary. This was mainly in terms of minor illnesses such as colds, dandruff and cuts (53%), and routine administration such as signing certificates for National Insurance (18%). Bridgestock[4] also found that the number of unnecessary consultations provided the least satisfying aspect of general practice for doctors.

The employment of a nurse as a front line reference and filter in general practice may be regarded in its negative aspect as making the doctor less accessible to patients. However, the evidence, including that derived from our study, strongly indicates that the majority of patients would not consider this to be of overriding importance. Practical considerations, such as greater efficiency in dealing reasonably quickly with large numbers of patients, easing the pressure on appointments systems and a ready source to patients of technically qualified advice from a nurse are likely to take precedence over the principle of first contact care by the doctor.

However, systems that work to the greatest all round satisfaction are generally those which can tolerate some degree of flexibility. Patients who expressly wish to see the doctor, despite the nurse's opinion that a consultation is not necessary, should not be obstructed. The basic element of choice should not be removed from the patient. For a few patients continuity and direct contact with their doctor is undoubtedly of paramount importance. This need may be in response to a particular incident or a consistent, strongly-held preference. Continuous periodic involvement with the doctor may well symbolize for some chronically ill patients the belief that they need not yet be resigned to their condition. These patients are likely to view the filtering role of a nurse as an intrusive element in their relationship with their doctor. In their study of attitudes of the public to para-medical services, Dixon et al.[14] found that employment of nurses in general practice was generally regarded with favour by their sample of 1,812. Of these respondents who objected (6%), fears were most often based on being unable to see the doctor when they wanted.

Continuity of care and the specialist

Patients' preference for direct access to a specialist, instead of by negotiation with the doctor, was also explored as an indicator of attitudes to the primary continuous care aspect in personal doctoring. We found that 201 (63%) of respondents would prefer to see their general practitioner before seeing a specialist. Ninety-six (30%) would like to be able to go direct to a specialist and 16 (5%) either did not know or said it would depend on the circumstances. Only seven (2%) had no preference. Patients' age, sex and social class were not significant variables. Cartwright[3] found that a much higher percentage of respondents would prefer to see a specialist via the doctor, (84%). It may well be that the difference between the figures reflects a growing tendency towards patients' preference for more autonomy in caring for their own health.

Of those who would prefer to go to a specialist via their general practitioner, most said they would rely on the doctor to confirm that the visit was necessary and to direct them to the best specialist. Many respondents' comments showed that they accepted this aspect of the general practitioner's role without question—"Getting the doctor's consent is the proper thing to do."

The main reason given by the 30% who would prefer to go direct to a specialist was that this would be quicker. This was in terms of cutting down the process leading to access to the specialist and getting to the root of the problem more quickly by drawing on his greater technical expertise. The second most common reasons given were to prevent the doctor blocking access to a specialist and so that the choice of specialist would not be determined solely by the doctor.

Few of our respondents appeared to consider the issue in its effect on the doctor/patient relationship in personal terms. When the relationship was mentioned, this was usually in general terms with regard to the doctor's loss of status and authority if the procedure of consulting him prior to seeing a specialist was omitted. This is illustrated by the following comments:

"Seeing your doctor first shows you are placing your confidence in him—he wouldn't like it if you went over his head."

"The doctor might lose confidence in the doctor/patient relationship you have if he thought you were going over his head."

"If you go over his head it's making out you've no time for your own doctor."

From the patient's perspective, the doctor's function as "middle-man" between specialist and patient appears to be a well established role expectation. As one respondent said: "That's what the doctor's there for." However, this function of the British general practitioner's role is a generalized expectation. It does not appear to be associated particularly with the relatively more intimate nature of personal doctoring.

Medical students in the consultation

The presence of a medical student or trainee doctor in the consultation removes to some extent the intimacy and privacy of the encounter. We assessed how much this mattered to patients by asking how they would feel if a medical student was present during consultation with the doctor. For Group A the question related directly to the forthcoming consultation, whereas for Group B it was entirely hypothetical. However, the responses of the two groups were closely matched.

The overwhelming majority of the sample, 285 (89%) said that they would not object to a student being present. Twenty-two (7%) said they would not like this and 13 (4%) said that they would not like a student to be present in some circumstances.

Women were more likely to prefer a student not to be present than men, $(p = <.05)$. One hundred and thirty-nine (95%) of the men said they would not mind this, but four (3%) would and three (2%) said that their attitude would depend on their reason for consulting. For the women, the figures were 152 (84%), 17 (10%) and 11 (6%) respectively.

Unmarried patients were also more likely to be concerned about a student being present than those who were married or had been married, $(p = <.05)$. Two hundred and nine (92%) of our married or previously married respondents would not object, 14 (6%) would and four (2%) said it would depend on circumstances. For those who had not been married, the figures were 76 (82%), seven (8%) and ten (10%).

Of the few respondents who voiced their preference to see the doctor alone, the reason most often given was that they might wish to discuss something "personal" or "private" with the doctor and they would be embarrassed by the presence of a third party. Some patients specifically mentioned having to undress for an examination in front of a student as a source of much embarrassment. This was the second most common reason for preferring to see the doctor alone.

General practitioners who are accustomed to having a trainee doctor or medical student in the room during consultations are quite likely to take their presence for granted. The Royal College of General Practitioners[1] point out that if a third party is present in the consultation he should be introduced to the patient and the reason for his presence explained. This is not just a matter of courtesy. By effecting this formal contact, the doctor recognizes that the norms of social intercourse still apply to the patient vis-a-vis the third party and implies that he understands the patient's reservations in relation to role expectations. Failure to acknowledge the needs of patients in this respect may be detrimental to doctor/patient relations and adversely affect the outcome of the consultation. One patient who had wanted to discuss her problem more fully with the doctor said:

> ". . . he had someone in. I don't know who it was, he didn't say. I didn't like it as I had to show my top. So I got out as quick as I could."

Another respondent failed to discuss the most important reason for her visit, a lump on her breast, because two students were present. It is open to conjecture whether she would have done so had an introduction and explanation been effected by the doctor.

Patients generally expect to see a general practitioner in a one-to-one consultation. This is an element in the set of expectations attached to the dynamics of general practitioner/patient role interaction which need not be confused with the more personal relationship implied in the concept of personal doctoring. Respondents' expressed attitudes to the presence of a medical student in the consultation gave no indication whatever that they regarded the presence of a third party to be intrusive in their relationship with the doctor. Those who expressed preference to see the doctor alone did so in relation to the expectations attached to his role, especially those of technical competence and affective neutrality, and the lack of these expectations attached to the student's role.

Whereas for many patients it was important that they had previously met the doctor they were about to consult, so that they knew what to expect, quite the reverse was so with regard to the hypothetical student. Patients said they would be considerably more embarrassed if they knew the student who was present. From the patient's perspective the medical student is in a state of transition; he has not yet acquired the role of doctor but is still learning the part. As one respondent explained her objection:

> ". . . it is because of the fact that he isn't qualified—that makes him just another person there, rather than just one doctor."

Generally, patients did not appear to be concerned about the presence of a medical student in terms of this affecting the intimacy and privacy of their encounter with the doctor. However, there are personal problems and conditions which some patients will have difficulty in discussing at all, much as they might like to. The presence of a third party, and the doctor's lack of under-

56

standing in dealing with this element, may considerably reduce the possibility that their reluctance will be overcome.

Personal problems

Patients' opinions with regard to whether they would discuss serious personal problems with their doctor or with someone else were assessed. Table 10 shows patient's first preference.

One hundred and sixty-three (51%) would talk to someone other than their doctor, 35 (11%) were not sure and 19 (6%) would not turn to anyone. One hundred and three respondents (32%) said that they would talk to their doctor. This result is close to Cartwright's finding of 28% who said that they might discuss a serious personal problem with their doctor.[3, p.107] In their comparative study of single-handed and partnership practices, Varlaam et al.[15] reported that 41% of patients registered with partnership practices had turned to their general practitioner for advice about personal problems.

Table 10

Who patients would talk to about a serious personal problem that was depressing them.

	%
Doctor	32
Relation/friend	27
Spouse*	15
Don't know	11
No one	6
Vicar/priest	4
Social worker	2
Others	3
Number (= 100%)	320

* Number in sample married = 177.

When we pressed respondents who had not mentioned the doctor as a first preference, whether they would consider talking to him about a serious personal problem, this percentage was increased to 56%. Table 11 shows responses.

Table 11

"Would you talk to your doctor about a serious personal problem?"

	%
Yes	56
No	37
Only if health affected	4
Don't know	3
Number (= 100%)	318

Table 10 probably reflects a more accurate picture of respondents' attitudes. Many respondents included in Table 11 who said that they would talk to the doctor, added a rider, for example: "Yes, but I would rather go to the social services as they are more helpful." "Yes, but I wouldn't waste his time."

57

There is some evidence that although patients may agree in principle that they would talk to the doctor about a personal problem, in practice they declined to do so when pressed by the doctor. In one such case the patient was consulting because of anxiety. The doctor asked if she knew what might be the cause and she said she did not know. However, when she was interviewed at home for the study it became quite obvious that she was well aware of the reason but, as she said: "I didn't like to tell the doctor." In this kind of situation neither doctor nor patient wins. The patient was not satisfied with the outcome of the consultation and expressed her resentment:

"He didn't tell me anything. Just gave me the prescription. He's writing out the prescription as he's talking to you. He just doesn't seem to listen."

The respondent's mother was also dissatisfied as she felt that the doctor should have questioned her daughter more persistently before prescribing Valium for her. The doctor, faced with resistance to his gentle probes and a waiting room full of other patients, perhaps felt that under the circumstances this was the best he could do.

Analysis of the comments of those who said they would not talk to the doctor about a serious personal problem shows that for most respondents the negative response was quite emphatic. The attitude of these respondents is in complete accordance with Parsons' definition of the doctor's role with regard to functional specificity, as described on page 9. This is aptly expressed by the following comment of one of our respondents:

"The general practitioner is not best qualified to deal with one's personal problems. He's not as well qualified as your next door neighbour."

Respondents often appeared even to resent the idea and were quite blunt in their reply. A common response was: "My personal problems are none of his business." This was the attitude of one young patient who made her opinion known to the doctor in no uncertain terms:

"Yeah, well OK then. Last week, not last week the week before, my mother came to see you. She's been going mad with her headaches, you know and that. And that's been getting us down as much as me mum. She says, 'Me head's killing,' and things like that. And she came to see you and, er, when she walked in you said to her, when she told me about it, 'What's up, have you had a row with one of your daughters?' I mean, me mother was quite upset about that. She's old-fashioned, you know. She doesn't think you tell your doctor things like this. And she was upset and she came home and told me. Dear God, you know! I mean, there and then I felt like coming down and seeing you, you know. I was blazing because you'd upset my mother . . . etc. and especially with someone being there. There was a student there as well. I mean she was really upset when she came home and she told me and that, well, you know."

This was part of one of the longest consultations over the study period, taking 16 minutes. About one-third of the consultation was taken up by the doctor explaining to the patient his reasons, in particular and in general terms, for enquiring into patients' personal problems. Such cases high-light the difficulties of doctors who take a holistic approach towards care of patients which is resisted by them. The patient in this case was not convinced by the doctor's reasoning and continued to regard his well-intentioned interest as unwarranted intrusion. She was nevertheless satisfied with the consultation because she was given the prescription she had come for.

However, not all patients who gave a negative response were quite so whole-hearted on the matter. Seventeen indicated that although they would not present their doctor with a personal problem, they would like to feel able to do so. Most of this group felt that their personal relationship with the doctor was not conducive to treating him as a confidante.

The data showed that patients of Dr. Y were more likely to discuss their personal problems with the doctor than those of Dr. X, (p = <.05). Sixty-two per cent said they would do so compared with 50% of Dr. X's patients. However, in practice the transcripts showed that patients of Dr. X more often talked to him about personal family and social problems. When they did so, it was usually at some length and in response to gentle probing openers. The number of years patients had been registered with their doctor did not appear to be a significant factor.

Social class was a significant factor in determining whether patients would talk to their doctor about a serious personal problem. Sixty-nine per cent of patients in Social Classes IV and V and 60% in Social Class III were likely to do so, compared with 30% in Social Classes I and II, (p = <.01). This finding is entirely consistent with that of other studies.[3,16,17] A review of the transcripts also bears out the evidence of the data. When personal problems were discussed in the consultation, with one exception, this was by Social Classes III, IV and V. Patients' problems were mostly concerned with inadequate housing and the effects on personal relationships of overcrowding. Difficulties experienced in employment or unemployment were also discussed. It may well be that the type of problems Social Classes I and II feel unable to cope with alone would more appropriately and profitably be taken to other professionals, such as a bank manager or lawyer.

There was a significant correlation between age and patients' attitudes in this respect, (p = <.05). We found that patients in the two age groups 25–44 and over 65 were most likely to discuss their personal problems with the doctor, 62% and 60% respectively. Fifty-six per cent of those in age group 45–64 said they would do so. It was the younger age group, 16–24, who were least likely to regard their doctor as a confidante, (46%). This finding is supported by Cartwright[3, p.109] who makes the point that the evidence is "contrary to the views aired by some doctors about the comparative dependency of the young." We found that it was the younger respondents who were most apt to be a little indignant towards the implied suggestion that their doctor might act as adviser and guide where problems other than those medical were concerned. This attitude was in direct contrast to the nostalgic comments of some older patients. The intensive person-centred style of Dr. Finlay, of radio and television fame, might be their ideal prototype of personal doctoring. As a 71 year old woman who had been registered with her doctor more than six years said:

"I wouldn't talk to the doctor about a personal problem. He wouldn't be interested. They're not like the old doctors who were part of the family almost. Times have changed."

59

Two basic approaches

1. Person-centred or illness-centred care. Although person-centred doctoring is certainly not confined to a relationship of continuous primary medical care by one doctor, it is an integral feature. As a measure of their attitude in this respect, we asked patients whether they thought the doctor's interest should be restricted to their medical condition or if he should also be interested in the patient as a person. The majority of our sample, 202 (63%) thought that their doctor should be interested in them as a person together with their medical condition. Comments of this group most often related to the observations that a person-centred, rather than a strictly clinical approach, was more likely to put patients at ease and elicit the type of personal information which was required at times to bring about better understanding of a condition. One hundred and twenty-two (32%) said that they expected the doctor to be interested only in their medical condition and 16 (5%) were not sure. Comments of some patients who elected for illness-centred care show that they did so with reservation and a practical outlook on the doctor's work load:

> "Doctors are there to treat you medically but if you had a more personal contact I think it would be more satisfying for the patient. There are more people than the doctor can give time to and the relationship isn't the same."

> "It is impossible to expect doctors to handle people as individual persons. The most you can ask for is medical competence."

We also asked respondents whether they felt that their doctor was interested in them as a person or not. Two hundred and five (64%) felt that he was, 61 (19%) thought he was not; 48 (15%) were not sure and 6 (12%) gave another response.

On the basis of whether the doctor would recognize his patient by name in the street and his knowledge of his patient's domestic situation, Cartwright[17, p.92] suggests that:

> " ... doctors have a rather less sympathetic and understanding relationship with their working-class patients."

Whilst accepting the limitations of the doctor population in the present study, the evidence does not support Cartwright's tentative finding. The vast majority of our respondents in Social Classes IV and V would discuss a personal problem with their doctor. They were also more likely to feel that the doctor's interest in them extended beyond a strictly clinical approach. Seventy-six per cent of those in Social Classes IV and V felt that the doctor was interested in them as a person, compared with 65% of Social Class III and 63% of Social Classes I and II, (p = <.05).

More patients of Dr. Y felt that he was interested in them as a person, 69% compared with 57% of Dr. X's patients. However, these figures could have occurred by chance in the sample, (p = <.10 > .05). It says much of Dr. Y's powers of communication that, despite the brevity of most of his consultations, an average of three minutes, he was clearly able to engender a sense of personal interest and rapport with his patients.

2. Impersonal, business-like or friendly style. Respondents were asked which kind of doctor they preferred: one who was impersonal and business-like, personal and friendly, or business-like but friendly. Two hundred and eight (65%) said that they preferred a business-like but friendly style. Ninety (28%) voted for a personal and friendly doctor. The impersonal and business-like approach was almost totally rejected. Only six respondents (2%) elected for this preference and 16 (5%) were not sure.

We also asked respondents who felt that they knew the doctor well enough to make such an assessment, what kind of relationship they had with him. Table 12 shows patients' preferred style of doctoring compared with their perception of the reality.

Table 12
Patients' preferred and perceived styles of doctor/patient relationship

Style of relationship	Preferred %	Perceived %
Impersonal and business-like	2	9
Personal and friendly	28	26
Business-like but friendly	65	59
Don't know/other	5	6
Number (= 100%)	319	271

Table 13
Marital status and patients' preferred and perceived style of doctor/patient relationship

Style of d/p relationship	MARITAL STATUS					
	single		married		previously married	
	prefd. %	percvd. %	prefd. %	percvd. %	prefd. %	percvd. %
impersonal or business-like	2	11	2	5	4	20
personal and friendly	26	12	26	29	36	36
business-like but friendly	71	66	66	61	50	42
don't know/ other	1	11	6	5	10	2
Number (= 100%)	93	77	176	149	50	45

Clearly, for the overwhelming majority of our respondents their doctor's style was in accordance with that which they preferred.

Marital status was a significant factor in determining respondents' perception of the relationship, ($p = <.01$). Table 13 shows patients' marital status and preferred style of doctoring compared with their perception of the relationship in reality. Single patients expressed the highest preference for a business-like but friendly approach (71%) and for 65% their preference matched reality. Of the 26% single patients who preferred a personal and friendly style, 14% felt that they did not have this warmer relationship. Preference and reality

61

corresponded most closely for married patients. There was also close correspondence for those who had previously married. This group was most evenly divided between their preference for the two styles of personal and friendly or business-like but friendly, 36% and 50% respectively. For only 8% did the preferred business-like but friendly style not match reality.

Only 24 patients of 271 thought that their relationship with their doctor was impersonal and business-like. This was most likely to be felt by patients who had previously been married and by those who were single, 20% and 11% respectively.

From their patients' perspective, the relationship style of the two doctors differed most markedly as far as the first two styles were concerned, (p = <.001). Seventeen per cent of Dr. X's patients felt their relationship with him was impersonal and business-like and 12% thought it was personal and friendly; whereas the figures were 2% and 38% for the patients of Dr. Y.

There do not appear to be any studies which attempt to relate patients' attitudes towards their doctor with measures of his personality. A sample of two general practitioners is obviously not appropriate and this is not attempted here.

It is a truism that communication is a two-way process and undoubtedly many variables contribute towards the outcome and impression of each snapshot of interaction. However, as far as the vast majority of our respondents were concerned, the basic tenor of their relationship with their doctor, as measured by these two basic approaches, was also likely to be their preferred style. It is not possible to assess the extent to which this consensus is a function of accommodation by patients to their doctor's style, or vice versa.

Interaction between doctor and patient is generally a matter of accommodation. Aspects of accommodation with regard to patients' expectations of the consultation are examined in the following chapter.

REFERENCES

1. Royal College of General Practitioners (1972). *The Future General Practitioner.*

2. Royal College of General Practitioners (1973). "Present State and Future Needs of General Practice." Third ed. *Report from General Practice* No. 16. *Journal of the Royal College of General Practitioners.*

3. Cartwright, A. (1967). *Patients and their Doctors.* London: Routledge and Kegan Paul.

4. Bridgestock, N. (1978). "Personal communication." A cohort of doctors in England and Wales who became unrestricted principals for the first time in 1969 was utilised. 884 doctors were assembled from information supplied by the Department of Health and Social Security. Of the 683 remaining in 1976, 439 responded to a questionnaire, of whom 216 responded to the section dealing with sources of satisfaction.

5. Hopkins, P. (1974). *Update, 8,* 348.

6. Clyne, M. B. (1974). "How personal is personal care in general practice?" *Journal of the Royal College of General Practitioners, 24,* 263.

7. Aylett, M. (June 1977). *Pulse,* p. 11.

8. Batty, J. (Aug. 1977). "Multiple G.P. Care Wins," *Pulse,* p. 6.

9. McKenna, M. S. and Wacker, M. D. (1976). "Do patients really want family doctors?" *New England Journal of Medicine, 295,* No. 5, 279.

10. Kaim-Caudle, P. R. and Marsh, G. N. (1975). "Patient Satisfaction Survey in General Practice." *British Medical Journal*, 262.

11. Gill, D. G. and Horobin, G. W. (1972). "Doctors, Patients and the State: Relationships and Decision-Making," *The Sociological Review, 20*, No. 4, New Series, 505.

12. Stimson, G. and Webb, B. (1975). *Going to See the Doctor*. London: Routledge and Kegan Paul, pp. 138–140.

13. British Medical Journal (1976). "Medical Manpower: How much can ancillaries take over?" Working paper by R. Klein and edited discussion. *British Medical Journal, 1*, 25.

14. Dixon, C. W. *et al.* (1975). "Attitudes of the Public to Medical Care: Part 5—Para-medical Services," *New Zealand Medical Journal, 82*, 5.

15. Varlaam, A., Dragoumis, M., and Jeffries, M. (1972). "Patients' opinions of their doctors—a comparative study of patients in a central London Borough registered with single-handed and partnership practices in 1969," *Journal of the Royal College of General Practitioners, 22*, 811.

16. Dunnell, K. and Cartwright, A. (1972). *Medicine Takers, Prescribers and Hoarders*. London: Routledge and Kegan Paul.

17. Cartwright, A. and O'Brien, M. (1976). "Social Class Variations in Health Care and in the Nature of General Practitioner Consultations," In *A Sociology of the National Health Service, Sociological Review Monograph* 22, Ed. M. Stacey: University of Keel.

CHAPTER VI

PATIENTS' EXPECTATIONS

One of the main aims of the research was to discover patients' specific expectations of their general practitioner in relation to a particular consultation and examine ways in which those expectations were met or altered during that consultation. Part of the questionnaire was also directed towards exploring aspects of communication.

Before proceeding to enlarge on the foregoing themes, the concept of expectations is analyzed in relation to the patients' perspective of the doctor/patient consultation. Patients' expectations with regard to five of the most commonly occurring management actions taken by the general practitioner are then examined. These are issuing sickness certificates for national insurance benefits ("sick notes"), prescribing, examining patients, taking or arranging tests and arranging referrals. We also attempted to assess how perceptive the doctor was in assessing the expectations of his patients in these respects. In relation to these specific expectations, the data and supporting evidence from the transcripts are drawn from the first part of the sample, the 160 respondents of Group A who were interviewed prior to their consultation with the doctor and again at their own homes to discuss what had transpired in the consultation.

In conclusion, factors which may adversely affect patients' ability to express their needs and expectations effectively to their general practitioner are identified. Data relating to this aspect are drawn from both Group A and Group B.

The concept of expectation

Expectation implies some definite grounds or reason for considering that an event or action is likely to happen. Hope is synonymous with expectation and adds the implication that the awaited event is wanted and/or desirable. The concept of expectations in relation to general practice has been analyzed effectively by Stimson and Webb.[1] Their linear model distinguishes between three types of expectation: background, interaction and action expectations.

Background expectations are derived from the individual's personal experience of encounters with general practitioners and incidents related by others. This aspect is essentially related to role theory, in that the patient's accumulated background knowledge enables him to play the part of patient according to the requirements of the basic doctor/patient interaction script. He knows what is expected of him and knows what to expect from the general practitioner.

Interaction expectations refers to "the process of presentation and decision making which leads up to the outcome". An alternative and perhaps more apt label may be "assessment expectations". Prior to consulting the doctor, the patient will have made his own assessment of the condition or problem. In relation to this, he will have consciously or subconsciously constructed expectations of the doctor's response and assessment. Patient and doctor view from different perspectives, which may be described as subjective lay and objective professional. Inevitably, occasions arise where the two assessment expectations are not in accord. For example, one of our respondents who had been consulting with hypertension and recurring conjunctivitis felt that the latter condition should have cleared up. The transcript shows his underlying concern which is contrary to the doctor's assessment of the condition.

Dr. "And how have your eyes been?"
Pt. "They've been a bit sore just lately. Like it was before you know. They felt as if I just wanted to put a pair of dark glasses on, you know, to comfort them like. It's er...."
Dr. "Have you been to see them at the Eye Hospital at all recently?"
Pt. "No."
Dr. "No. They discharged you about three years ago, didn't they?"
Pt. "Yes."
Dr. "Mm ... let's have a look."
Pt. " 'Course I retire in September."
Dr. "Uh huh. What are you going to do then?" (A discussion about the patient's retirement plans follows whilst blood pressure is recorded.) "That's O.K. Thank you."
Pt. "I was thinking of, er, going to the Eye Hospital again, you know. But I thought I'd just see how they go on like."
Dr. "There's no need."
Pt. "No?"
Dr. "No, they're doing all right."
Pt. "Are they?"
Dr. "Mm."
Pt. "Oh."
Dr. "So you want some more drops and you want some more tablets."
Pt. "Capsules and tablets, yeh."

Action expectations follow closely upon assessment. These are the specific actions which the doctor is expected to take in his management of the condition. In the above case the patient had expected to be referred to the Eye Hospital. Having been assured that this was not necessary, he was given a prescription instead. Action expectations may be sub-divided into ideal and actual expectations, i.e. the action that the patient would like the doctor to take and the action which he thinks will be taken. Interaction of ideal and actual expectations in conflict is clearly illustrated by one of our respondents who said:

> "I hope he will give me a sick note but I don't think he will. It's always reduced to either he does or he doesn't."

In order to distinguish between these two types of action expectations, we asked patients what they wanted the doctor to do and whether this was also what they expected to happen. With regard to prescriptions, ideal and actual expectations were matched for 104 (65%) respondents. For 35 (22%) there was some mismatch of the type described above and for 21 (13%), expected action, whether ideal or actual, was an unknown quantity for the patient. The figures were similar with regard to the expectation of being examined by the doctor but showed an increase in uncertainty attached to the expectation of having tests carried out or being referred for a specialist's opinion. For the majority of patients, the action they wanted the doctor to take was synonymous with the action they expected would be taken in the management of their condition. Wants and expectations are therefore used interchangeably, unless otherwise indicated.

Certificates

Expectations of receiving a certificate were well in excess of Cartwright's finding of 9%.[2, p.28] Thirty-four (33%) of our respondents had this expectation, 66 (64%) did not and three (3%) were not sure. Fifty-seven of our respondents were not eligible to receive sickness certificates for national insurance benefits.)

Dr. X was less likely to issue certificates, ($p = <.01$). He did so at ten (13%) of his consultations, whilst Dr. Y did so at 26 (33%). Certificates were issued to 36 (35%) patients: 15 were first certificates, 19 intermediate and two were final certificates. The doctors' perception of their patients' wants was most accurate in this respect. They assessed that 31 (30%) patients expected to receive a certificate. Only five of the 34 patients who had wanted a certificate were not indicated on the doctor's record form as having this expectation. Conversely, the doctors assessed that two patients had wanted a certificate when, according to the patient, this was not expected.

With regard to correspondence of expectation and action: only three patients who had wanted a certificate were not given this. In only one of these cases was the patient disappointed by not getting the expected first certificate, the other two already had intermediate certificates which had not lapsed. For those who had not expected or did not know whether to expect a certificate, only five were given.

Prescriptions

In their report of trends in general practice, the Royal College of General Practitioners[3] estimated that in a typical year a general practitioner would see 600 patients with coughs and colds, 325 with skin disorders, 300 suffering from depression and anxiety, 100 with chronic rheumatism, 50 with high blood pressure, eight with heart attacks, five with strokes, five with cancers and five with acute appendicitis. Patients received an average of six prescriptions each per year and the largest groups of drugs prescribed would be tranquillizers, sleeping pills and antibiotics. Studies in Britain and the United States have estimated that within a given period of twenty-four to thirty-six hours, between 50–80% of the adult population would have taken one or more "medical" drugs.[4,5]

Interviews for the present study were carried out at the doctors' surgeries from June to September. Of the 160 patients taking part in the study, the most commonly occurring diagnosis related to psychological disturbance, (Figure 2). Prescriptions were issued to 121 of the 160 respondents, (76%). Psychotropic drugs were most often prescribed, followed by analgesics and antibiotics. A total of 169 items were prescribed.

The doctors' prescribing habits appeared to be very similar in that Dr. X wrote a prescription at 62 (78%) of his consultations and Dr. Y at 59 (74%). There was very little difference between the two in the numbers of repeat prescriptions issued. A single item was prescribed on 100 occasions, two items on 16 occasions and more than two items on five occasions. Seventy-six (45%)

Figure 2 Diagnoses made by diagnostic category. (210 diagnoses involving 160 patients)

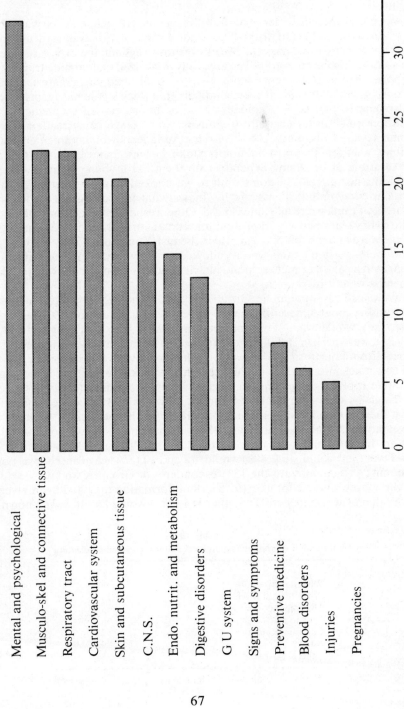

67

of those items were for medication which the patient had used previously. This figure is well below an estimated 75% for repeat prescriptions given to adults.[6]

We found enough evidence to show that people are inclined to be wary about the content and effect of drugs. This is not surprising in view of growing public awareness of possible harmful effects of many drugs and the exposure given to this subject by the lay media. The now fully publicized thalidomide tragedy and reports on the birth control pill have probably had the greatest effect in arousing public distrust. It seems unlikely that Illich's polemic against clinical iatrogenesis, that is the "epidemic" of conditions caused by medical intervention which in turn require treatment, would leave many readers without some sense of disquiet.[7] Most of our respondents who commented on this subject said that they just did not like taking drugs. Some explained that they were afraid of becoming dependent on them. As a young woman with pre-wedding nerves said: "I don't want to get hooked up on anything." Another patient commented: "I assume he knows what he's doing but I sometimes wonder. I think we're all guinea-pigs." Other respondents said that they would like to have more information about the content of prescribed medication, and some were in the habit of asking their chemist. The unusual view expressed by one man—"I don't think you're allowed to know what you're taking," was repeated by another male respondent who said: "You aren't allowed to ask the chemist what it is."

We asked respondents in Groups A and B whether they liked to be told something about a prescription they were given by the doctor. 193 (60%) said that they would want some information. Those who said they did not, 75 (24%), were perhaps taking it for granted that directions for using would have been given. Fourty-six (14%) were satisfied to leave to the doctor the decision of how much information should be given. Only six (2%) were not sure or gave another reply. Age, sex and social class were not significant variables.

Table 14 shows the items of information which 193 respondents indicated that they would like to be given about prescribed medication. We asked these respondents whether, on the basis of past experience, they would expect to be given this information by their doctor. One hundred and thirty-three (69%) said that they would, 46 (24%) would not and 14 (7%) gave another response. Looking at the reality for the 121 respondents of Group A who were actually given a prescription: for 111 (92%) the information they had been given by their doctor was sufficient. The other ten (8%) would like to have known the

Table 14
Information wanted by respondents about prescribed medication

	%
What it is for	99
What effect it will have	70
The contents	65
How to take	60
Contraindications	52
Name	20
Other	8

Number of respondents = 193

68

content and effects of the medication. Ten patients did not know the purpose of the medication, of whom two said they would like to know. Clearly, for almost all of our respondents the doctor correctly assessed how much information to impart to his patient.

Looking at the doctors' perception of their patients' expectations, we found that the doctors assessed that 78 (49%) of our respondents expected to receive a prescription. From a nationwide sample of 453 unrestricted principals, Stimson[8] showed that four out of five doctors estimated that in 80% of their consultations the patient expected a prescription. Comparing this finding with Cartwright's [2, p.28] figure of 52% who expected a prescription, Stimson draws the tentative conclusion that most doctors overestimate their patients' expectations. In Stimson's analysis of his data the doctors were divided into three groups: high, medium and low estimators of patients' expectations. Our two doctors came well within the low estimators category. The doctors in Stimson's low estimators group assessed that 0–79% of patients expected a prescription. In the present study the doctors' total estimate of their patients expectations was 78 (49%). It appears that, besides being low estimators, they were also underestimators as 96 (60%) of our respondents actually expected a prescription. Twenty-six (16%) patients who had wanted a prescription were not judged to have been expecting this by their doctor. Conversely, the doctors assessed that seven of their patients wanted a prescription, although this expectation was not indicated by these respondents in the pre-consultation interview.

In Cartwright's study the respondents were asked what they "thought or hoped the doctor might do for them" during a consultation which had occurred up to two weeks previously.[2] Fifty-two per cent expected the doctor to prescribe for their condition and 71% said that they were actually given a prescription. In the present study patients were asked in the pre-consultation interview whether they expected to be given a prescription. After the consultation they were asked whether a prescription had been issued. Ninety-six (60%) said that they expected to be given a prescription for at least one item, only four of whom were disappointed. Fourty-four (28%) did not expect to receive a prescription and 20 (12%) did not know what to expect. Eighteen and eleven patients respectively in each of these two groups were given prescriptions.

The case histories of the four patients who wanted a prescription but were not given this by the doctor, illustrate how patients' expectations and attitudes may be affected by what transpires in the consultation.

Respondent 006

A 34 year old lorry driver was consulting about vague "aching all over" which the doctor diagnosed as "anxiety". He said that he was very worried about the condition. Irritability and depression were having a serious effect on his every day life. He just wanted the doctor to repeat the prescription for Valium and increase the dose. The doctor's consultation record showed that he was aware that his patient was very worried although he considered this was not appropriate. He did not assess that a prescription was expected on this occasion. There was no indication in the transcript of what the patient wanted. Instead of just being given the prescription he expected, our respondent was

69

given an intermediate certificate and referred to a specialist for investigation. In the post-consultation interview he said that he was even more worried than before because of the unexpected referral and added—"There must be something wrong if he's sending me to a specialist."

Respondent 093

A 54 year old construction labourer was consulting with pains across his shoulders. He said that he was not worried and just wanted the doctor to examine his shoulders and give him a prescription. He wanted to be able to get back to work as being at home was making him irritable and depressed, but expected that he would get a sick note. The doctor indicated that a prescription had not been expected and that the patient appeared to be more worried than was appropriate. The consultation transcript shows that the patient appeared to be reluctant to say what he had come about and the doctor was equally reluctant to take up the cues that his patient offered:

Dr. "And how are you Mr. X?"
Pt. "Well I'm a bit better."
Dr. "Good."
Pt. "Yes."
Dr. "Yes. Anything troubling you now at all?"
Pt. "Well, it still troubles me at night, but not as much as it was doing though."
Dr. "No, good. So it's a lot better? Hm?"
Pt. "Yes, it's er well on the mend, yes."
Dr. "Good. Yes, oh well that's fine, and what is it you've come to see me about today?"
Pt. "Well it's not, you know, quite. . . ."

The expected examination was made and certificate given. But it was a "bit of a shock" for our respondent when the doctor said that the trouble may be caused by the chest and that this should be investigated. The doctor's assessment of how worried the patient was appears to be accurate. Although the respondent had said he was not at all worried about the condition, in the post-consultation interview he said:

> "I'm a lot less worried. I'm hoping after the X-rays they'll be able to find out what's wrong and treat it."

Respondent 104

Yet another reaction to an unexpected action by the doctor was shown by a 68 year old company director who was consulting about a swelling in the groin. The condition was having a "very serious" effect on his everday life as the pain made walking difficult. He was not at all worried and just wanted to be examined and given a prescription. The patient's expectation of receiving a prescription was not indicated on the doctor's record form and, again, the patient was considered to be more worried than seemed appropriate to the doctor. An examination was made and referral to a surgeon advised. Although our respondent's expectations were changed from wanting a prescription to anticipating an operation, he said that he felt neither more nor less worried and the consultation had been very worthwhile. As he said:

> "I'm going to get something done about it."

70

Respondent 106

This was the patient's first consultation with Dr. X and was a relatively long counselling session in which marital, family and employment problems were discussed. The transcript is incomplete as the tape came to an end in what seemed to be mid-session after 18 minutes. The patient, a 33 year old clerk typist, was consulting because she felt tense and had "trouble with nerves". She wanted to be examined and given a prescription and sick note. The condition appeared to be having quite a serious effect on her everyday life but she said she was not worried about it. From a medical and social point of view she considered the condition to be "quite serious". She felt irritable and depressed and was unable to manage her work, run her home and cope with her young son alone. Early in the consultation she hinted to the doctor that she wanted a repeat prescription for Valium. When the doctor appeared to ignore this and asked about her work our respondent returned with a stronger hint:

Pt. "The doctor gave me some Valium last week and they . . . . Actually I don't know if they were too strong but oh I was dopey for about 4 days, really dopey, you know. They did slow me down of course."

Dr. "Mm hm."

Pt. "My old doctor, whom I had when I was bad when I was ill about Easter time, gave me something. Could it be called Seneril, or Sera something? They didn't seem to have any effect, except they did calm me down a bit. They didn't make me feel absolutely dopey."

Dr. "Now tell me about your past health. What illnesses have you had?"

The consultation record shows that the doctor diagnozed an "anxiety state" which he described as serious socially but not medically. He was aware that his patient wanted a prescription but not that she also expected to be examined and given a sick note. He obliged with the latter only. Our respondent appeared to be very appreciative nevertheless and considered the consultation to have been very worthwhile:

"He's explained more fully how I can go about helping myself to sort out my problem."

As in the case of Respondent 093 referred to above, this respondent had said prior to the consultation that she was not at all worried. Again, the doctor's assessment of this appeared to be more accurate as she now said she was far less worried. Her pre-consultation expectations were met in only one respect, i.e. the certificate, but in the post-consultation interview she said there was nothing else she now required.

In Balint's terms, the doctor himself may be the most potent drug which he prescribes. However, this particular prescription takes a great deal longer in the writing. The above consultation may almost have been designed to illustrate the broad thesis that if doctors had more time to give to their patients, less tranquillizers would be prescribed. Or, the more doctors are able and willing to give of themselves, the less necessary it is for them to give medication. Dunnell and Cartwright[4] asked their sample of general practitioners whether they would give fewer, more or the same number of prescriptions if they had more time to spend with each patient. Fifty-two per cent thought that they would write fewer prescriptions and 47% thought their prescribing habits would not change. Only 1% thought they would write more prescriptions.

It seems quite likely that the length of time given to the above consultation would play havoc with the time schedule of most general practitioners. Such cases may well point the need for a separate counselling service within general practice, so that the unscheduled counselling consultation does not inconvenience doctors and patients by disrupting appointments systems. However, there are at least three problems here. Firstly, many general practitioners may feel that they require a relatively long counselling session with their patient before they come to a decision with regard to prescribing psychotropic drugs initially. Secondly, spontaneity would be lost in the progression of establishing the expectation of receiving a prescription for tranquillizers and discussing with the patient the reasons behind this need. Thirdly, the act of referring the patient for counselling might well increase her anxiety.

During the study period Dr. X conducted six counselling consultations in which intimate details of the patients' personal problems were discussed. In five of these cases the patient was described by the doctor as being in an "anxiety state". Tranquillizers were prescribed for four of these patients. In each case our respondent said that the consultation had been worthwhile. Two expressly mentioned that they felt better for having spoken to the doctor. Expectations had been met for all but Respondent 106 referred to above.

Satisfaction for one of these six respondents was clearly based on expectations and doctor's actions being in accord. A 28 year old woman said that she was "desperate" about her condition and stressed that if the doctor did not give her Valium, which she said had been previously prescribed by another doctor, she would change her doctor. In the post-consultation interview she said:

> "I take back what I said about him yesterday. So long as I get my prescription for tablets I like him."

The implication being that if her expectation was not met, then her opinion of the consultation might be quite different.

There was some evidence in the transcripts that both doctors attempted to educate their patients into an awareness that tranquillizers can only be a temporary solution to personal problems and that stress is a normal part of the pattern of life. One of these instances was a classic case of pre-wedding nerves.

Respondent 036

Pt. "I think it's my nerves because I'm getting married in a few weeks."
Dr. "Have you had your bowels open?"
Pt. "Yes."
Dr. "All right?"
Pt. "Yes."
Dr. "Good. Well, that sounds a very reasonable proposition, doesn't it. Well, I'm very pleased to hear it, aren't you?"
(Long pause.)
"Em, what sort of pains are you getting?"
Pt. "Like butterflies."
Dr. "Butterflies in the tummy, yes?"
Pt. "Mm."
Dr. "Very common. Has everyone told you that? Oh dear. Well, it's a normal response isn't it really, to anybody who's embarking upon some new

situation in life. Whether it's marriage, or a job, or going overseas for something. Changing your way of life. Do you feel you need something for it? Because if you feel that you know what it is and you can cope with it, then I'd rather not give you anything. But if you feel it's so bad as to cause you problems, then I'll give you something."

Pt. "Mm."
Dr. "I think it's.... I think when you know what it is ..."
Pt. "Yes."
Dr. "And you get a bit worked up, a bit churned up, and you think, oh well it'll all be over, you can deal with it. If you don't know what it is—and I'm sure you're right ... I'm not giving you anything. See how you go on. But if you really feel you need something, you can always came back and see me."

This patient had not known whether she wanted a prescription from the doctor or not but she was quite worried and wanted to be examined. The doctor indicated that she had expected only reassurance, and reassure her he did. She came away from the consultation less worried and was convinced that the condition she had thought to be "quite serious" medically, was not so in fact. The consultation was altogether worthwhile in spite of her expectation not being met. She was also satisfied with the doctor's decision not to prescribe for her on this occasion.

Respondent 143

The educative value of her doctor's advice was not as effective in this case. The patient was a 46 year old coffee bar attendant who wanted a repeat prescription for Valium. She assessed that her condition was "serious" in medical terms and "very serious" socially but she said that she was not worried about it. The doctor considered that the condition was not serious in either respect but that his patient appeared to be very worried. On the evidence of the transcript, this last estimate appears to be more accurate. Our respondent was not at all convinced by the doctor's advice that the dosage of tablets she had been taking for anxiety was so small that they would have very little effect and she should therefore try to do without them. In the face of her expectation being thwarted, the patient used two strategies in an attempt to sway her doctor's action in favour of her expectation. The first was to gently dissolve into tears. There followed a kindly but determined attempt by the doctor to elicit some cause for his patient's apparent distress, apart from not being given what she wanted. However, he met with no success and apparently decided to resolve the problem for the moment by prescribing a placebo:

Dr. "Right. (Pause) I'll give you something slightly different."
Pt. "Give me the same tablets, doctor, 'cause etc."
Dr. "Beg your pardon?"
Pt. "Give me the same tablets as I was on 'cause they were the only things as was ever any good to me."
Dr. "Mm."
Pt. "They were great. I would prefer you wouldn't change them."
Dr. "Well, I think you'd better leave it to me to decide what you should have, don't you?"

It was at this point that the patient turned to a second strategy which we had noted in several transcripts where it seemed that fulfilment of expectations was threatened. This was quoting what the "other doctor" had said or done in support of an expectation of the same action being taken again.

Pt. "Well, I'd prefer to go back to the other place, 'cause they told me if ever I had any problems to go back to them. 'Cause etc. I would always go back there."

Dr. "Which other place are you talking about?"

Pt. "XX College. They told me if ever I had any problems to go back to him, you know."

Dr. "XX House you mean?"

Pt. "Yes, I'd prefer the other tablets if you will give them to me, but you know, I've felt great up to this last fortnight. Honest to goodness, I feel great, you know."

Dr. "Mm hm."

Pt. "I prefer you wouldn't change them, you know."

Dr. (Pause) "Now, you have a go with these, taking one a day like you did before etc."

In the post-consultation interview the above respondent launched a tirade against the doctor, which she would no doubt like to have delivered to him directly had this not been precluded by the norms of doctor/patient interaction. She made her dissatisfaction with the consultation very clear, adding: "I always thought he was a good doctor before this." The relationship between thwarted expectations and dissatisfaction with a consultation is very clear in the cases described on pages 65 and 71 and Respondent 143 above. For such patients satisfaction with the doctor may be only as good as the met expectations of his last performance. The lady's own performance during the above consultation was interesting in its range of paralinguistic effects. These fluctuated from a persuasive display of genteel distraction to unconcealed anger in the space of less than two minutes, as it became obvious that her expectation of being prescribed Valium was going to be thwarted.

The prescription is, of course, not merely a written order for medication: as with the sick note it also confers legitimation of the sick role upon the recipient. For some patients the ability to sustain this role may be an integral part of their personal relationships. A spirited attempt to defend such a position may well result in the face of threat.

Clinical examinations

Looking first at our doctors' perception of their patients' expectation: they assessed that 39 (24%) of their patients expected to be examined. This underestimate was quite considerable, in that 81 (51%) said that they expected to be examined at the forthcoming consultation. Fifty-five (35%) said they did not expect this and 23 (14%) were not sure. Of the 81 who wanted to be examined, the doctors were aware of the expectation in 33 cases. Six patients were perceived as having wanted to be examined, although this expectation was not indicated to the interviewer.

Our respondents appeared to set almost as much store on being examined as they did on being given a prescription. Their expectation is well in excess of

Cartwright's finding of 23% who reflected that they had expected to be examined.[2, p.28] Of the 98 (61%) patients in our sample who were examined by the doctor, 67 had expected this, 21 had not and ten had not known what to expect.

Patients who had expected a prescription were more likely to have this expectation fulfilled. Fourteen of our respondents who had expected to be examined were not. Of those 14, 12 thought that the consultation was worthwhile, five of whom said that they were less worried about their condition after being reassured by the doctor. However, in two of these cases the patient considered the consultation to have been a waste of time for both herself and the doctor.

Respondent 041

A 60 year old home help was consulting the doctor with "nerves". The only expectation she had indicated in the pre-consultation interview was to be examined. Because the doctor did not examine her she considered that he had not been sufficiently thorough. Perhaps the true source of her dissatisfaction was shown in the post-consultation interview, when she said that she would like to have asked the doctor to prescribe Librium and to discuss her housing problem with a view to obtaining his support for a change of council house. The only reason she gave for not referring to these matters in the consultation was that she did not know the doctor well enough. However, elsewhere in the interview she had said: "I can't seem to say what I want."

Respondent 142

This 61 year old woman consulted with the expectation of having her neck examined, with reference to a recent car accident, and having her blood pressure checked. Neither of these expectations were fulfilled. The doctor recorded that she had expected a prescription only. She was very worried about her neck, which the doctor did not realize. This is hardly surprising, as she appeared to be quite satisfied with the doctor's assurance that all was well:

Pt. "Could you tell me Doctor X, is it all right that my neck clicks now and then?"

Dr. "Yes."

Pt. "Is that all right?"

Dr. "Yes, it may do. Yes."

Pt. "Fine. Thanks."

She continued to express her concern to the interviewer:

> "The doctor just asked if my neck was all right and dismissed it, although I would like to have discussed it—the pain I'm having. I mean, I don't know if it's all right."

She was also very concerned that her blood pressure had not been taken. Apparently a doctor whom she had seen previously had said that it should be taken every three months and this was the main reason for consulting. Although he considered this quite unnecessary in her case, if the doctor had realized the extent of her concern, he may have made this simple check in order to reassure her. In these circumstances there is little or nothing the patient can do to aleviate her concern, except to acquire faith in the doctor's judgement.

Of the 21 patients who had been examined but had not expected to be, almost all were less worried about their condition and considered the consultation to have been worthwhile. Only one respondent was more worried as a result of the consultation.

Respondent 103

A 79 year old respondent was consulting with pain in her stomach. She expected to be given a prescription and a urine test to be made. She reluctantly agreed to be examined and the doctor discovered a small urethral caruncle which needed to be cauterized. In the post-consultation interview she said:

"I certainly didn't expect him to say this, I had the shock of my life."

In this case the patient thought the doctor had been too thorough and she did not agree that the referral was necessary. The expectation of a visit to hospital caused much concern and she expressed doubts about taking her doctor's advice in this respect. The doctor appeared to be quite unaware of her concern and indicated that his patient was not at all worried.

Investigations

The doctors in our study underestimated their patients' expectations of having investigations carried out. Twenty-six (16%) respondents wanted to have investigations carried out, 97 (61%) did not and 36 (23%) were not sure. The doctors assessed that only 2% expected investigations.

Investigations were arranged or carried out during the consultation for 37 (23%) patients. Eleven patients who had expected to have tests taken were disappointed. One of these was Respondent 142 referred to above, who was so concerned about having her blood pressure taken. The transcript shows that she asked directly for the test to be done. This we found to be rather unusual. In two further cases where the expectation of having an investigation carried out was not met, the patient's attitude and expectations were clearly altered during the course of the consultation. One was a 46 year old patient who was consulting about symptoms which she had taken to be the start of the menopause. She had been very nervous about consulting as she was afraid that the doctor would not be sympathetic. She also wanted a cervical smear test to be arranged. In the post-consultation interview she said she was "amazed" that the doctor had taken so much trouble: "He didn't make me feel a freak." She was fully reassured about her condition and the advice that a repeat of the smear test was not yet necessary. She was less worried and said that the consultation was very worthwhile.

In the second of these two cases, an expected test for anaemia was not arranged for our 23 year old respondent who was suffering from nausea and tiredness. The doctor's remarks that she was the third person he had seen that day with such symptoms and that it seemed to be a virus infection, convinced and reassured her. She said that she was less worried now that she knew the condition was not serious and she considered that the consultation was worthwhile.

Of the 97 patients who had not expected it, investigations were arranged for 14. Eight of the 36 patients who had not known what to expect had tests arranged. Patients did not appear to be worried by having tests taken unexpec-

76

tedly; almost all said that they felt less worried and the consultation was worthwhile. Seven of these unexpected cases were the measurement of blood pressure.

X-ray investigation/referral

Referral for X-ray investigations or to a specialist in hospital were the actions least expected by our respondents and least often taken by the doctor. Fourteen (9%) people said that they wanted to be referred. This figure of 9% corresponds closely with Cartwright's finding of 6% who wanted to be referred.[2, p.28] One hundred and twelve (70%) of our respondents did not want to see a specialist and 33 (21%) were not sure. The doctors under-estimated their patients' expectations at nine (5%). Of the 14 who expected a referral, the doctors indicated that only six had expected this. Two patients who did not want to see a specialist were thought by the doctor to have this expectation.

Twenty-one (13%) patients were actually referred, compared with Cart-wright's finding of 10%. Of those 21, five wanted a referral, seven did not and nine were not sure. Contrary to expectations, patients did not appear to be worried by an unexpected referral. In each case, except for a patient who was referred to the Eye Hospital and Respondent 103 referred to above, these respondents said that they were either less worried or felt the same.

As far as concordance of expectations and action was concerned, there appeared to be a case for "ask and it shall be given". Of the 14 patients who wanted a referral, five asked and were referred, nine did not ask of whom one was referred. One respondent who had firmly expressed his intention to ask for a barium meal X-ray barely hinted at this in the consultation:

"You don't think it could be ulcers do you doctor?"

The others gave the doctor no indication of what they wanted.

Communication of expectations

A comparative view of the expectations given by respondents in the pre-consultation interview and the consultation transcripts says much of the doctor/patient relationship. We found that although many patients appeared to be quite sure of what action they wanted the doctor to take, they very rarely asked him for this directly. When asked: "What can I do for you today?" patients invariably responded with a description of their complaint which was tantamount to a plea for action. They may have known exactly what they wanted but consistently responded to the general notion of—"It's not up to me to tell the doctor what I want." For example, a 66 year old man wanted to be examined, have tests carried out and be referred to a specialist. Having given him the initiative, the doctor promptly regained control and dispatched his patient and his expectations in 40 seconds. The transcript is reminiscent of Szasz and Hollender's ideal type activity/passivity model which is associated with the parent/infant relationship.[9]

Dr. "George X. How are you today?"
Pt. "About the same as last week, doctor. It's er . . . I'm taking the tablets, but er . . ."

Dr. "Well, you've got to persevere."
Pt. "Yes."
Dr. "Did I invite you for a flu injection?"
Pt. "Yes."
Dr. "Have you got enough tablets for another week?"
Pt. "Yes, for another week."
Dr. "Well, we'll give you another sick note . . ."
Pt. "Yes."
Dr. ". . . and we'll see you in another week."
Pt. "The lady doing interviews is coming to see me on Monday afternoon."
Dr. "Make your appointment for next Friday afternoon, not in the morning."
Pt. "Friday afternoon. Right doctor."
Dr. "O.K.?"
Pt. "O.K. Yes, thank you."
Dr. "O.K. chief."
Pt. "Right. Bye-bye."
Dr. "Bye-bye."

The aura of mystique and authoritarianism which is commonly attached to even the most simple actions taken by a doctor may work to the detriment of the patient. For example, an anecdote related by one of the doctors in the study described an occasion when one of his patients consulted accompanied by her mother. The doctor prescribed tablets for the daughter, as he had done over the years many times. On this occasion the mother advised him that her daughter had never been able to take tablets. The doctor expressed his surprise that this apparently articulate young lady had never told him this herself and had simply not used the prescribed medication.

One of our respondents was consulting for a repeat prescription for the oral contraceptive pill. She also expected to be examined for adverse side effects and have her blood pressure taken. Although she was clearly concerned about possible harmful effects of the pill, she failed to broach this with the doctor and continued to worry about it. She thought that the doctor had not been thorough enough because the waiting room was so full of people he was not prepared to spend more time with her.

This example was repeated in another consultation. One respondent wanted to be examined and seemed to have been given a cue to ask for this:

Dr. "And how have you been getting on?"
Pt. "Great. Fine thanks. No problems."
Dr. "No problems?"
Pt. "No."

There was no indication in the post-consultation interview why she had not talked about her worries.

There appears to be a built-in deference on the part of patients towards doctors which inhibits the normal course of communication. How much of this is a function of doctors' self-perceived status in relation to their patients and *vice versa* is impossible to determine. From comparative observation of our respondents in the interviews and recordings of the consultations, a chameleon effect was much in evidence. We had observed this in the pilot study and had, therefore, added questions into the main study which might determine the cause of the change in many patients when they were confronted with their doctor.

All respondents in Group A and Group B were asked if they ever felt nervous about seeing their doctor, using the term in the generally accepted sense of being uneasy or agitated. Over a quarter of our sample, 88 (28%), said that they often or always felt nervous. Only 42 (13%) said that they occasionally did and 190 (59%) said that they never did. The correlation between this factor and social class was not significant. There was a very significant correlation between the variable and sex. We had anticipated that women would feel more at ease in communicating with their doctor. This assumption was based on evidence that their attendance rates are higher and those who had brought up a family would be likely to have had more continuous, meaningful interaction with their doctor. However, we found that the reverse was the case. Women were far more likely to anticipate a visit to the doctor with some unease. Ninety-one (51%) said that they felt nervous, compared with 39 (28%) of the men. Thirty-nine (43%) of the women and 14 (36%) of the men said that they always felt nervous, $(p = <.001)$.

We also found that respondents in age group 16–24 seemed most likely to be uneasy. Forty-one (54%) said that they felt nervous about a visit to the doctor compared with 30 (33%), 44 (40%) and 15 (35%) consecutively in age groups 25–44, 45–64 and over 65, $(p = <.05)$. However, when we extended this question by asking how often our respondents felt like this, we found an inverse correlation. Forty-six (78%) of those over 45 years old said that they always or often felt nervous about seeing the doctor, compared with 18 (60%) and 24 (59%) in age groups 25–44 and 16–24, $(p = <.05)$.

Of the 305 respondents who were registered with one of the two doctors in the study, those of Dr. X were more likely to feel apprehensive about consulting. Sixty-nine (47%) said that they felt nervous, compared with 53 (33%) of Dr. Y's patients, $(p = < .05)$. There is little doubt that this finding is affected by the different styles of receiving patients at the two practices, as described in Chapter IV.

Table 15
"Why do you often/always feel nervous about seeing the doctor?"

	%
(a) Respondent's temperament	32
(b) Awe of doctors in general	22
(c) Unknown outcome of a visit to doctor	17
(d) Doctor's manner	12
(e) Embarrassment re certain conditions	7
(f) Don't know	7
(g) Doctor may not be sympathetic	2
(h) Difficulty in explaining symptoms, etc.	1

n = 88 respondents (14 giving 2 reasons)

We asked respondents who had said that they were always or often nervous why this was. Table 15 shows responses. From the patients' perspective, 36% of the problem appears to be doctor-centred, (items (b), (d) and (g)), and 33%

79

patient-centred, (items (a) and (h)). Comments relating to "respondent's temperament" largely concerned patients' increased anxiety because of having to wait to see the doctor and fear that he may think that their reason for consulting was not serious enough to warrant consulting. These patients attributed their worry to their own temperament but obviously their problems were, in a sense, partially doctor-centred. With regard to the category "awe of doctors in general", one young person's comment was particularly articulate and represented the general sense of other remarks:

> "They're in a position of authority. They have power over you and know everything about medicine. I don't know anything."

Doctors and patients inevitably view the presented condition from very different perspectives. Patients' expectations will obviously be affected by their view of how serious their condition or problem is. We asked both doctors and patients to make their assessment of the presented condition in both a medical and a social sense. Table 16 shows their comparative responses. Judging by their doctors' assessment, some patients appeared to under-estimate the medical seriousness of their condition and a few to over-estimate this. Many patients, 38%, said that they did not know whether their condition was serious or not. This uncertainty would undoubtedly affect patients' approach to the consultation and gives support to the view expressed in the Journal of the Royal College of General Practitioners.[10]

> "Of all the possible encounters with different professionals, few are more threatening to a person than seeing a doctor. Some symptoms are potentially serious, many appear so, and most consultations engender some anxiety for the patient."

Table 16
Doctors' and patients' perception of the seriousness of presented condition medically and socially

	very serious	serious/ quite serious	not serious	don't know	Number of patients (= 100)
Medically	%	%	%	%	
Doctors	4	26	70	0	151
Patients	7	16	39	38	146
Socially					
Doctors	11	42	47	0	151
Patients	15	51	28	6	146

With regard to the effect of the condition on patients' everyday life; the patient is clearly in a better position to make this assessment. Judging by their estimate, the doctors did not appear to appreciate the extent of their patients' problems from a social point of view. Fifteen per cent of the patients considered that their problem was having a very serious effect on their everyday life, 42% a serious or quite serious effect and 28% said it was not serious. The doctors' assessment was 11%, 51%, and 47% consecutively.

The above findings show some empirical support for the premise that there is divergence between the perspectives of doctor and patient which is likely to affect communication between the two.

Recognizing that patients are generally apprehensive about visiting their doctor, the Patients' Association has advised their members how to go about explaining their problem to the doctor. This advice includes the suggestion that patients should make a list of their problems and symptoms, with dates, and think about what they intend to say.

Most of our respondents felt that talking to their doctor was always easy, 184 (68%). However, for quite a large group this basic element of communication presented some problem. Eighty-two (30%) said that talking to the doctor was sometimes or always difficult; 6 (2%) were not sure. There appeared to be no relationship between social class and difficulty experienced by patients in this respect.

The correlation between sex and this variable was very significant. Seventeen (11%) of the women said it was always difficult to talk to the doctor, 40 (26%) said it was sometimes difficult and 96 (63%) found it always easy: whereas only 3 (3%) of the men always had difficulty, 22 (19%) sometimes and 88 (78%) found communication easy in the consultation, ($p = < .01$). Three patients of each sex were not sure.

Talking to the doctor was more likely to present problems for younger patients. Fourty-seven (37%) of those aged between 16–44 said this was always or sometimes difficult, compared with 35 (25%) of those over 44 years old, ($p = < .01$).

Two hundred and fifty-three of the respondents who were registered with one of the two doctors in the study gave responses to the question of how easy it was to talk to him. Sixty-two (52%) of Dr. X's patients said this was always easy, 41 (35%) found communication sometimes difficult and 15 (13%) said it was always difficult. The figures for Dr. Y's patients were 113 (84%), 20 (15%) and two (1%), ($p = < .001$).

We were able to identify the main reason why patients found it always or sometimes difficult to talk to the doctor. Contrary to expectation, ignorance of medical terms did not appear to be the main factor, although this possibly contributed to difficulty in explaining symptoms. Table 17 shows the main problems which affected our respondents. Only 39 respondents are represented in both Table 15 and Table 17. It would, therefore, appear that we have identified two variables which are to some extent distinct.

Most of the patients who commented regarding "doctor's manner" were drawn from Group B. Almost all of these respondents' remarks referred to the doctor being unapproachable, for various reasons. It is not possible to assess the extent to which this may affect therapy from the data in this study.

Table 17
"Why do you find it sometimes/always difficult to talk to the doctor?"

	%
(a) Doctor's manner	52
(b) Difficulty in explaining symptoms etc.	25
(c) Respondent's temperament	8
(d) Awe of doctors in general	6
(e) Embarrassment re certain conditions	6
(f) Other	3

n = 82 respondents (6 giving 2 reasons)

Of the 22 respondents who said that they had difficulty in describing how they felt to the doctor, few had any additional comment to make. Looking at the transcripts, however, there were many cases in which this factor was apparent. Examples follow:

1. Pt. "These last four weeks I've been getting these pains . . ."
   Dr. "Mmm. The heat doesn't help with these . . ."
   Pt. "The bone feels as if it's stiffening, you know."
   Dr. "Yes. Will you try some tablets?"

2. Dr. "What was the pain like when it came on?"
   Pt. "It was a weight."
   Dr. "A weight?"
   Pt. "Here."
   Dr. "Was it a gripping pain?"
   Pt. "Oh, I don't know—right in my back etc. Into behind my ears and somewhere in my throat."

3. Dr. "Do you get any pain when you pass water?"
   Pt. "No. It's just a weird feeling."
   Dr. "Mm?"
   Pt. "It's a weird feeling."

4. Dr. "Yes? What's the sensation in your leg?"
   Pt. "It's something like somebody screwing the muscle and then as they release it, it's like a pack of needles going in."
   Dr. "Is it a painful feeling then?"
   Pt. "I wouldn't say painful. It's sort of . . ."
   Dr. "Is it a numb feeling then?"
   Pt. "Oh killing, it's killing."
   Dr. "Is it a *numb* feeling?"
   Pt. "Er, well, I must get a bit of numbness in it because I had it one day from 3 o'clock."
   Dr. "But do you feel that the sensation is different when you touch it?"
   Pt. "Well, I get . . . No, I just have to hold it like that."
   Dr. "Well, when you touch it like that, does it seem as though the sensation in that part of the leg is diminished—when you touch it?"
   Pt. "I kept walking up and down and kept going round and round. I had it from 3 o'clock one day."

In the last example, the doctor's frustration is just as apparent as that of his patient. Both gave up the unequal struggle to elicit and provide the required information. Knowledge of medical terms would undoubtedly help patients to describe the location of their problem or pain. But giving verbal expression to subjective bodily sensations is another matter. No two people will experience a sensation or approach it in exactly the same way. There are no well-defined base lines by which individuals can measure and describe pain and discomfort.

It has been said that in the last analysis, the quality of medical care depends on the quality of interaction between doctor and patient.[11] Communication is the essence of any relationship or encounter. The Royal College of General Practitioners[10] remind doctors that:

"... a patient often faces his doctor feeling physically weak and emotionally upset ... Such vulnerability creates a corresponding responsibility for doctors—both individually and collectively, to understand their patient's fears and feelings, and their difficulties in expectation and communication."

These fears and feelings are well expressed by one of our respondents:

"Doctors and medicine are such an unknown area to the average person one tends to over-react. When I see them, it means I'm not in the best of health and I don't feel as capable as my usual self. I worry if it's serious and unknown."

REFERENCES

1. Stimson, G. and Webb, B. (1975). *Going to see the Doctor*. London: Routledge and Kegan Paul, p. 28.

2. Cartwright, A. (1967). *Patients and their Doctors*. London: Routledge and Kegan Paul.

3. Royal College of General Practitioners. (1977). *Trends in General Practice*.

4. Dunnell, K. and Cartwright, A. (1972). *Medicine takers, prescribers and hoarders*. London: Routledge and Kegan Paul.

5. White, K. *et al.* (1967), "International Comparisions of Medical Care Utilization," *New England Journal of Medicine. 277*, 516.

6. Dunnell, K. (1971). "Medicine Takers and Prescribers". *In* Parish, P. A. "The Prescribing of Psychotropic Drugs in General Practice," *Journal of the Royal College of General Practitioners, 21*, Supplement No. 4.

7. Illich, I. (1976). *Limits to Medicine*. London: Calder and Boyars.

8. Stimson, G. (1975). "General Practitioners' estimates of patient expectations, and other aspects of their work." Medical Sociology Research Centre, University College of Swansea, Occasional Paper No. 3.

9. Szasz, T. and Hollender, M. H. (1956). "A contribution to the Philosophy of Medicine," *Archives of Internal Medicine, 97*, 585.

10. Editorial, Patient Power. *The Journal of the Royal College of General Practitioners* (1974), *24*, 138.

11. Korsch, B. M. and Negrete, V. F. (1972). "Doctor-Patient Communication," *Scientific American, 227*, 66.

CHAPTER VII

CONCLUSION

Interaction between doctor and patient is an exercise in communication. The effectiveness of the interaction will depend, as in all other face to face encounters, on the ability of the participants to make contact and clarify their expectations, be they implicit or explicit.

The present study shows that the doctor/patient interaction is a particularly sensitive process. The patient, often under stress, has difficulty in articulating her needs and the doctor, often under pressure, may have difficulty in perceiving his patient's expectations.

From the moment the patient initiates the process of "going to see the doctor" the interaction mechanism is at work. Patients can easily be inhibited by receptionists whose role is often seen as a barrier, preventing ready access to the doctor. Evidence from this and other studies shows that preliminary enquiries from qualified nurses about the patients' illness or problems are not likely to be resented. Such queries from receptionists may be very much resented. On the whole, there were few complaints about receptionists in the present study. However, there does appear to be a need for further studies in this field. The extent of the "funnel/filter" role of the receptionist should be explored, together with the reaction of patients to these roles. It may be unrealistic to assume that receptionists are not required to assess the need for appointments or visits. Consideration might be given to training which would equip receptionists, at the least, to be aware of symptoms which indicate the necessity for rapid attention. The whole area of receptionist/patient/doctor interaction may repay further research, the emphasis of which should be upon the patient/practice interaction, rather than the patient/doctor interaction.

The way in which the patient is actually received by the doctor can have a direct effect on the quality of a consultation. The mechanistic system of light signals, buzzers and coloured discs found in some group practices may produce an alienating effect which reduces both doctor and patient to different cogs in the same machine. The simple acts of showing a patient out and welcoming another in by name are gestures of resistance to the automation of human relations.

A related and more basic barrier to effective interaction lies in the status attitudes of doctors and patients, as perceived in relation to themselves and to each other. There is some indication that younger general practitioners and trainees are abandoning the often over-rigid formality of their elders. In a society which is better educated, certainly in a social sense, and which is also more egalitarian in attitude, if not in economics, it is increasingly inappropriate for social interaction to take place on the basis of superior/inferior stances. Doctor and patient are moving towards the same end, i.e. to facilitate the return of the latter to health or optimum capacity. Conditions which produce the minimum anxiety in the consultation will clearly promote this aim. Such conditions will undoubtedly include removal of out of date status barriers on the part of the general practitioner.

In our study women found it more difficult to communicate with their male doctor and were more apprehensive about the prospect of a consultation. It is

84

generally acknowledged that women see a doctor more often and with relatively more intimate conditions. Yet, general practice and all other branches of medicine continue to be male dominated. Theoretically, since sexual equality became law, discrimination in selection of medical students does not take place. However, it is likely that a cultural lag will ensure that the current approximation of one-third female medical students will continue for some years. The number of women doctors in active practice may also be affected by the difficulties arising from the inevitable career interruption associated with rearing a family. Meantime, the effect of a lack of women doctors on female patients can only be a matter of speculation. Many patients of Dr. Y said that they preferred to see the lady doctor of the practice for gynaecological conditions. One woman in our study said she had first noticed a vulval cyst two years previously. Although she was afraid that this might be malignant, she had not consulted a doctor as there was no female general practitioner at Practice X. There is a need for studies of this specific aspect of doctor/patient relationships.

An interesting finding of this study is that patients may not set as high a value on personal doctoring as is assumed by the profession itself. Doctors tend to have an idealized perception of themselves as a "friend of the family", taking a paternalistic view which they feel is welcomed by their patients. In fact, whilst many people, especially the young, favoured a more friendly approach, they did not necessarily want a traditional personal doctor but rather one who was business-like and competent. In some cases any indication of pastoral interest on the doctor's part was positively resented, especially by patients who were his educational and social peers and the young. Also, it may well be that younger patients are inhibited in presenting more intimate conditions and problems to a "friend of the family" doctor. Many patients in our study appeared to value the affective neutrality of interaction with the doctor, rather than the personal aspects of the relationship. This area of the doctor/patient relationship should be clarified by further study, bearing in mind the implications for management of general practice.

Failing to meet patients' expectations can be a further barrier to effective interaction. For some patients satisfaction with a consultation will be a reflection of the extent to which their expectations have been fulfilled. Patients may have firmly established expectations, whether for simple measures such as a blood pressure check or for something more emotive such as tranquillizers. Thwarted expectations did on occasion lead to dissatisfaction but by no means always. As would be expected, the degree of dissatisfaction appeared to be in direct correlation with the strength of the expectation. The most emotional reactions came from patients who were not given a prescription for tranquillizers which they had expected. (Declining faith in religion may have paved the way for technology in the shape of tranquillizers to fill the vacuum, certainly only 4% of our sample would consider talking to a clergyman about their personal problems.) In such cases as this the meeting of patients' expectations is not necessarily good therapy on the doctor's part. It is, however, important that the doctor explains his reasons for not meeting expectations. Patients may not always appreciate his views but when the matter is discussed and advice or alternative action is recommended, satisfaction for the patient is more likely to follow than if the subject is dismissed out of hand.

The patients in this study appeared to have a realistic set of expectations. Of 313 expected actions only 41 (13%) were not met. Much has been written about doctors submitting to pressure from patients, especially when pre-scribing. However, our evidence shows that with regard to the five manage-ment actions discussed, see Chapter VI, the two doctors consistently under-estimated patients' expectations.

In order to appreciate more fully the patients' perspective, doctors need to be more aware of the fear of illness and its disruptive nature in their patients' daily lives. There was evidence in our study that the latter aspect was also underrated by the doctors. In a Report of the Working Party on Primary Medical Care[1] it was recommended that:

"All doctors, whatever their specialty, should possess some knowledge of the ways in which personality and social factors influence the response of their patient to disease and to its treatment or prevention."

This report also points out that:

"Much of the ill-health dealt with by general practitioners stems from the failure of individuals to make appropriate adjustment to their life situa-tions."

There is certainly evidence of this in the present study.

In order to alleviate problems caused by possible communication barriers in the doctor/patient relationship as outlined in this conclusion, it would seem to be necessary, above all, for general practitioners to adopt their patients' perspective. From that viewpoint the doctor's own role can be re-assessed. In this re-assessment there should be a place for the application of the skills of the behavioural sciences. It is through an understanding of the processes of interaction and social problems associated with illness that a fruitful doctor/patient relationship is most likely to be established.

REFERENCE

1. "Report of the Working Party on Primary Medical Care." (1970). British Medical Association Planning Unit Report No. 4.

Appendix 1   Pre-consultation questionnaire for Group A.

Year of b/sex: _____ 1 2   3 4   5 6   m/f

Registration: Dr. X/Y/other   <1 year 1–3 years 3–6 years 6–9 years 9 years+
                   1   2   3   1   2   3   4   5

Birth place: _____   1   2   3   4   5

Res. U.K.:   <1 year   1–5 years   6–10 years   10 years+   life
                1   2   3   4   5

Mar. status: single   married   widowed   sep.   div.
                  1   2   3   4   5

Completed ed: 14   15   16   17   18   18+
                  1   2   3   4   5   6

Occupation: (prev. if retired) _____
                 of husb. (prev. if decd.) _____
                 1   2   3   4   5   6   7 (student)   8 (unemployed)

Religion: C/E RC J   JW   CS   Meth.   Hdu. Mos. none
               1   2   3   4   5   6   7   8   9
               other _____ 11

1. When did you last consult a doctor at the practice?
   never   1
   <1 week   2
   1 week–1 month   3
   1 month–3 months   4
   3 months–6 months   5
   6 months–1 year   6
   1 year–2 years   7
   2 years+   8

2. Have you ever wanted to see the doctor before the earliest
   appointment offered to you?
   no   1
   don't remember   2
   first time attender   3
   yes: 4
       occasionally   1
       often   2
       not if urgent   3

3. How helpful do you find the receptionists when you are making
   an appointment?
   very helpful   1
   quite helpful   2
   receptionists vary   3
   don't know   4
   other (state)   5
   not helpful (probe)   6

4. Did the doctor ask you to make this appointment?
   yes   1
   no:
        respondent   2
        spouse   3
        relative   4
        friend   5
        social worker   6

5. If you found that the consultation was to be with another doctor instead of the one with whom you have an appointment, how would you feel about it?
   would not matter   1
   would depend on circumstances (probe)   2
   would not accept it (probe)   3
   would not like it (probe)   4
   other   5

6. Are there any circumstances when you would not wish a medical student to be present during a consultation?
   no   1
   don't know   2
   yes (probe)   3

7. In these circumstances would you ask the doctor to see you by himself?
   yes   1
   don't know   2
   no (probe)   3

8. When you see the doctor today a medical student may be present. How would you feel about this?
   would not mind   1
   would not like it (probe)   2

9. Is there a doctor at the practice whom you think of as your doctor?
   yes (probe)   1
   no   2

10. Do you think your relationship with Dr. . . . . (given above) is (prompt)
    impersonal and business-like   1
    personal and friendly, or   2
    business-like but friendly?   3
    don't know   4
    other   5

11. How well do you think Dr. . . . . (given above) knows you?
    very well   1
    quite well   2
    not very well   3
    not at all   4
    don't know   5
    other   6

88

12. Do you think that talking to Dr. .... is (prompt)

     always easy   1
     sometimes difficult, or   2
     always difficult?   3
     don't know   4
     other   5

13. Why do you think this is?   1

14. Do you think the doctor's interest in you should be

     (a) restricted to your medical condition, or that
     (b) he should also be interested in you as a person?
        (a)   1
        (b)   2
        don't know   3
        other   4

15. From past experience of your doctor/doctors, do you think that he does/they do take an interest in you as a person?

     yes   1
     don't know   2
     other   3
     no (probe)   4

16. How important to you is this particular visit to the doctor?

     very important   1
     quite   2
     not very   3
     don't know   4

17. Do you feel nervous about seeing the doctor today?

     yes:
        very   1
        quite   2
        a little   3
     no   4
     don't know   5

18. Why do you think this is?   1

19. Have you prepared in your mind what you will say to the doctor when you go in to see him?

     yes/more or less   1
     no   2
     other   3

20. What have you come to see the doctor about today? (prompt— "is there anything else?")

     (IF MORE THAN ONE REASON, ASK WHICH IS MAIN REASON AND MARK "p", "s" and "t")   1
           2
           3

     (IF MORE THAN ONE MEDICAL AND/OR SOCIAL REASON GIVEN, ASK ABOUT EACH IN TURN THROUGH TO AND INCLUDING Q30).
     (IF NO MEDICAL CONDITION/SOCIAL PROBLEM)   1

21. How long have you been seeing Dr. X/Y about this complaint/problem?

	p	s	t
first time	1	1	1
less than 2 weeks	2	2	2
2 weeks–1 month	3	3	3
1 month–3 months	4	4	4
3 months–6 months	5	5	5
6 months–1 year	6	6	6
1 year+	7	7	7
don't know	8	8	8

22. How long have you had the condition/been aware of the problem?

less than 1 week	1	1	1
1 week–2 weeks	2	2	2
2 weeks–4 weeks	3	3	3
1 month–2 months	4	4	4
2 months–4 months	5	5	5
4 months–1 year	6	6	6
1 year+	7	7	7

23. Have you seen any other general practitioner about it?

yes (probe)	1	1	1
no	2	2	2

24. Why are you not seeing Dr. . . . . (given for 23) about it this time?

	1	1	1

25. Did you take any action regarding the condition or treat it yourself before coming to see the doctor about it?

	p	s	t
yes (probe + source of advice)	1	1	1
no	2	2	2
could not	3	3	3
don't remember	4	4	4
yes:			
chemist	1	1	1
medic.	2	2	2
non-medic.	3	3	3
self	4	4	4

26. Why did you decide to treat the condition yourself rather than see the doctor about it?

	1

27. In a medical sense, how serious do you think your condition/problem is?

very serious	1	1	1
serious	2	2	2
quite serious	3	3	3
not serious	4	4	4
don't know	5	5	5

28. Thinking of the effect of this on your everyday life, how serious
    would you say it is?

very serious	1 1 1
serious	2 2 2
quite serious	3 3 3
not serious	4 4 4
don't know	5 5 5

29. In what way?   1

30. How worried are you now about the condition/problem?

very	1 1 1
quite	2 2 2
not very	3 3 3
not at all	4 4 4
don't know	5 5 5

*"Now I would just like to ask you briefly what you want the
doctor to do for you today."

31. Do you want the doctor to give you a prescription today?

no	1
don't know	2
yes:	3
1. new	1
2. repeat	2
1+2.	3

32. Do you expect he will give you a prescription?

yes:	
all	1
not all (probe)	2
no: (probe)	3
don't know	4

33. Do you want the doctor to examine you today?

yes (probe)	1
no	2
don't know	3

34. Do you expect that he will?

yes	1
no	2
don't know	3

35. Do you want the doctor to take any tests today, or arrange for
    any tests to be taken?

yes (probe)	1
no	2
don't know	3

36. Do you expect that he will?

yes	1
no	2
don't know	3

37. Do you want the doctor to arrange for you to go for any investigations or arrange for you to see someone else?

yes (probe)	1
no	2
don't know	3

38. Do you expect that he will?

yes	1
no (probe)	2
don't know	3

39. Do you want the doctor to give you a certificate today?

yes:	
first	1
intermediate	2
final	3
first and final	4
no	5
don't know	6

40. Do you expect that he will?

yes:	
first	1
intermediate	2
final	3
first and final	4
no	5
don't know	6

41. Is there anything (else) you want the doctor to do for you today?

don't know	1
no	2
other (state)	3
yes:	4
1. medical:	
(a) advice	1
(b) reassurance	2
2. social:	
(a) advice	1
(b) reassurance	2
3. result of investigation	1
4. check on progress	2
5. diagnosis:	
(a) from doctor	1
(b) confirmation	2
6. immunization/vaccination	4

42. Do you expect that he will do this?

yes	1
no (probe)	2
don't know	3

43. Do you think that the doctor will ask to see you again about this condition/problem?

	p	s	t
yes	1	1	1
no	2	2	2
don't know	3	3	3

Appendix 2.

Letter explaining the aims of the study for Group A

Dear

  The enquiry which you have agreed to take part in is being carried out by us at the above address. With your help we hope to find out more about patients' needs and expectations in connection with their general practitioners. Your opinions on this matter are extremely important as it is the view of the patient, rather than the doctor, which forms the major part of our study.

  We assure you that the information which you have already given and whatever you say in the second interview, will be completely confidential to the research team. A number allocated to you by the research team will appear on the questionnaires instead of your name. This will ensure that neither your doctor nor anyone else will be able to identify your part in the research.

  We feel sure that the results of the enquiry will be of value both to patients and their doctors. However, without your help the project would not be possible.

  I look forward to seeing you again at your home on _____.

Yours sincerely,

Appendix 3   Post-consultation questionnaire for Group A.

"First of all I would like to ask you some general questions and then talk about your last visit to the doctor."

1. Could you tell me which kind of doctor you would rather
    have—one who is (prompt)

impersonal and business-like	1
one who is personal and friendly, or	2
one who is business-like but friendly?	3
don't know	4

2. Is there any doctor you would prefer to see instead of the
    doctor you saw yesterday/today?

yes (probe)	1
no	2
don't know	3

3. If you had a serious personal problem which was depressing
    you and you wanted to talk to someone about it, who do you
    think you would turn to?

spouse	1
relation	2
friend	3
vicar/priest	4
social worker	5
tutor	6
other	7
would not turn to anyone	8
would depend on circumstances	9
don't know	10
doctor (code 4/1)	11

93

4. Would you talk to your doctor about a personal problem?
    yes   1
    no   2
    don't know   3
    other   4

5. Why is that?   1

6. If you attended the surgery about a minor illness or injury
   would you, or would you not, be satisfied if a nurse attended to
   you instead of the doctor?
    yes   1
    don't know   2
    other   3
    no (probe)   4

7. If you wanted to see a specialist and the present system was
   changed so that you could choose between going to him
   directly, or going through your doctor as we have to now, which
   would you prefer to do?
    prefer G.P. (probe)   1
    prefer specialist (probe)   2
    depends on circumstances   3
    don't know   4
    other   5

8. When you see the doctor about a troublesome condition, do
   you, or do you not, like him to explain what the condition is?
    yes   1
    no   2
    would leave it to doctor   3
    depends on condition   4
    don't know   5
    other   6

9. How full do you like his explanation of a condition to be?   1

10. From past experience of your doctor/doctors, how full do you
    think his/their explanation of a condition would be?   1

11. When the doctor gives you a prescription do you, or do you not,
    like him to tell you something about it?
    yes   1
    yes, if new to me   2
    would leave it to him to decide   3
    no   4
    don't know   5
    other   6

12. What do you like to be told about a prescription?
    don't know   1
    name   2
    content   3
    form   4
    what it is for   1
    how it will affect me   2
    contra-indications   3
    how to take it   1
    other   2

94

13. From past experience of your doctor/doctors, do you think you would be given this information or not?

    yes:
        all   1
        not all   2
        if one asks   3
    no   4
    depends on circumstances   5
    don't know   6

14. If the doctor were to arrange for you to have an investigation, e.g. an X-ray, or arrange for you to see someone else, would you want him to explain why it was necessary, or not?

    yes   1
    no   2
    would leave it to him   3
    don't know   4
    other   5

15. From past experience of your doctor/doctors, do you think this would be explained to you, or not?   1

16. If the doctor had not told you something you wanted to know during a consultation, do you think you would ask him about it, or not?

    yes   1
    no   2
    might   3
    don't know   4
    other   5

17. Why do you think you might not ask him?   1

18. Do you ever feel nervous when you are seeing the doctor?

    never   1
    yes: 2
        always   1
        often   2
        occasionally   3

19. Why do you think this is?   1
    * "Now I would just like to ask you a few questions about your general health."

20. Do you have any condition which you have consulted the doctor about in the past but which you no longer expect him to help you with?

        yes (probe)   1
        no   2

21. Have you any condition or illness which you are continuing to see Dr. .... about?

        yes (probe)   1
        no   2

22. Would you describe this as a long term or a short term condition?

    long term   1
    short term   2
    don't know   3
    other   4

23. How long have you been seeing him about it?
          <1 month   1
          1 month–3 months   2
          3 months–6 months   3
          6 months–1 year   4
          1 year–2 years   5
          2 years–4 years   6
          >4 years   7

24. Apart from this/During the past four weeks have you had any illness, injury, pain or discomfort which you have not seen the doctor about?
          yes (probe)   1
          no   2
          don't remember   3

25. Have you taken any action or treated the condition (given for 24) in any way?
          yes (probe + source of advice etc.)
               a. medical   1
               b. non medical   2
               c. self   3
               d. chemist   4
          no   5

26. Can you say why you did not go to see the doctor about it?   1

27. During the last four weeks have you suffered from
          (a) severe depression or tension, or from
          (b) abnormal tiredness or
          (c) sleeplessness
          which you have not seen the doctor about?
               yes:
                    (a)   1
                    (b)   2
                    (c)   3
               no   4

28. Are you still troubled by this?
          yes   1
          no   2

29. Have you had any advice about it from anyone?
          yes (probe + source of advice etc.)
               a. medical   1
               b. non medical   2
                 a. + b.   3
          no   4

30. Did you follow this advice?
          yes   1
          no   2

31. Did the advice help with the .... (given for 27)?
          yes (probe)   1
          no   2
          don't know   3

32. Apart from this/Have you (a) taken any action or (b) treated the condition yourself?
    yes
      (a)   1
      (b)   2
      (a) + (b)   3
   no   4
   don't remember   5

33. Do you think this helped?
    yes (probe)   1
    no   2
    don't know   3

34. Do you think the doctor would have been able to treat the condition (given for 27)?
    yes   1
    no   2
    don't know   3

35. Why did you not go to see him about it?   1

36. Do you know what it was that may have caused the .... (given for 27)?
    yes (probe)   1
    respondent declined to answer   2
    no   3

37. Do you think the doctor might have been able to help you with this/these problem(s) (given for 36)?
    yes   1
    no (probe)   2
    don't know   3

38. Why did you not go to see him about it?   1
    * "Now I would like to ask you about your visit to the doctor today/yesterday."

39. Do you think the consultation was long enough for you to say everything you wanted to the doctor?
    yes   1
    no (probe)   2
    don't know   3

40. When I saw you before, you said you wanted to see the doctor about .... Did you talk to him about this/each of these?
    yes:
      all   1
      not all (probe)   2
    no (probe)   3

41. Did you talk about any other problems while you were with the doctor? (prompt "anything else")
    yes (what)   1
    more than one   2
    no   3
    don't remember   4

(IF *NEITHER* A MEDICAL CONDITION NOR
SOCIAL PROBLEM)   a.   1
(IF REQUEST FOR B.C. PILL ONLY)   b.   2
(IF *ALL* SOCIAL, RATHER THAN MEDICAL)   c.   3
(IF MORE THAN ONE CONDITION/PROBLEM, ASK
ABOUT EACH IN TURN THROUGH TO AND
INCLUDING Q49)

42. When you saw the doctor today/yesterday about ....
    did he tell you anything about your condition?

                                                   p s t
        yes (probe)   1 1 1
        said nothing was wrong   2 2 2
        no: 3 3 3
            awaiting test results   4 4 4
            had insufficient information   5 5 5
            was not necessary   6 6 6
            could not   7 7 7
        other (state)   8 8 8

43. Did you expect him to say this?
        yes   1 1 1
        no   2 2 2
        don't know   3 3 3
        other (state)   4 4 4

44. Do you agree with the doctor?
        yes   1 1 1
        no (probe)   2 2 2
        don't know   3 3 3
        other (state)   4 4 4

45. Did you tell the doctor that you did not agree with him about it?
        yes   1 1 1
        no   2 2 2
        don't remember   3 3 3
        other (state)   4 4 4

46. Can you say why you did not tell him?   1

47. Was there any information or advice about p/s/t that you would
    have liked from the doctor?
        yes (probe)   1
        no   2
        don't know   3

48. Why did you not ask the doctor?   1

49. How serious did the doctor seem to think .... was?
        very serious   1 1 1
        serious   2 2 2
        quite serious   3 3 3
        not serious   4 4 4
        don't know   5 5 5
        other (state)   6 6 6
    (IF MORE THAN ONE MEDICAL CONDITION
    REPEAT BACK TO 42)

98

50. During the consultation, did the doctor examine any part of
    your body?
        yes (prompt "Anywhere else")   1
        no   2
        don't remember   3

51. Did you think this was necessary?
        yes   1
        no (probe)   2
        don't know   3
        other (state)   4

52. During the consultation did the doctor take any tests or arrange
    to have any tests taken?
        yes (probe)   1
        no   2
        don't remember   3

53. Do you think that this was necessary?
        yes   1
        no (why not)   2
        don't know   3
        other   4

54. During the consultation, did the doctor arrange for you to go
    for any investigations, or arrange for you to see someone else?
        yes (probe)   1
        no   2

55. Did he explain why he was recommending (see 54) . . . .
        yes (probe)   1
        no   2
        don't remember   3
        was not necessary   4
        other   5

56. Did you want him to explain why it was necessary?
        yes   1
        no   2
        don't know   3

57. Did the doctor give you a prescription?
        no   1
        yes: 2
            (a) new—1 item   1
                    2 items   2
                    >2 items   3
            (b) rpt—1 item   1
                    2 items   2
                    >2 items   3

58. What did the doctor tell you about the prescription?
        told nothing   1
        1. name   2
        2. content   3
        3. form   4
        4. what it is for   1
        5. how to take it   2
        6. what effect it will have   3
        7. contra-indications   1

99

59. Could you tell me what condition(s) the prescription is for?
        yes (probe)   1
        don't know   2

60. Is there anything (else) you would like to know about the prescription?
        yes   1
        no   2
        don't know   3
        other   4

61. What would you like to know about it?
    1. name   1
    2. content   2
    3. form   3
    4. what it is for   1
    5. how to take it   2
    6. what effect it will have   3
    7. contra-indications   1

62. Could you say why you did not ask the doctor for this information during the consultation?
        did not occur to me at the time   1
        did not want to bother the doctor   2
        don't know   3
        other   4

63. Is there anyone else you might ask for the information who would be likely to tell you?
        yes (who)   1
        no   2
        don't know   3

64. Have you taken the prescription to the chemist yet?
        yes   1
        no   2

65. Did you ask the chemist anything about the prescription?
        yes (probe)   1
        no   2
        don't remember   3

66. Do you think you will take/use what the doctor has prescribed?
        yes   1
        no (why not)   2
        don't know   3
        other   4

67. Was there anything (else) which you would have liked the doctor to prescribe for for you?
        yes (what)   1
        no   2
        don't know   3
        other   4

68. Could you say why you did not ask for this?
        yes (probe)   1
        no   2

69. Did the doctor ask you to make another appointment?

	p	s	t
yes (probe for which condition)	1	1	1
no	2	2	2
return at own initiative	3	3	3

70. Did the doctor give you a certificate?

yes:
(a) first		1
(b) intermediate		2
(c) final		3
(a) + (c)		4
no		5

71. Did the doctor give you any other advice or instructions during the consultation today/yesterday?

yes	1
no	2
don't remember	3

72. What did he say? 1

73. Do you think you will follow this advice?

yes	1
no	2
don't know	3
might	4
other	5

74. Why do you think you will not/might not? 1

75. How do you feel about the doctor's thoroughness in dealing with p/s/t?

	p	s	t
very thorough	1	1	1
sufficiently thorough	2	2	2
don't know	3	3	3
other	4	4	4
not thorough enough	5	5	5

76. In what way do you think he has not been sufficiently thorough? 1

77. Was there anything the doctor said during the consultation that you did not really understand?

yes (probe)	1
no	2

(IF RELEVANT (see pre-cons. 30)—ask 78/skip to 81)

78. Do you think the doctor really understood how you felt about the condition/problem?

yes	1
no (probe)	2
don't know	3

79. When I saw you before, you said that you were—very worried/quite worried about .... Do you think that the doctor realized you were?

yes/think so	1	1	1
no/don't think so (probe)	2	2	2
don't know	3	3	3
other	4	4	4

80. Why do you think this was?
    don't know   1
    did not show concern   2
    other   3

81. As a result of seeing the doctor today/yesterday, do you feel
    more worried, or less worried than you were before the
    consultation?
    less   1 1 1
    more   2 2 2
    same   3 3 3
    don't know   4 4 4

82. How interested did the doctor appear to be in you and your
    condition?
    very interested   1
    quite interested   2
    not (probe)   3
    don't know   4
    other   5

83. Is there anything else that you would like to have discussed
    with the doctor?
    yes (probe)   1
    no   2
    don't know   3
    other   4

84. Why did you not ask the doctor about this?   1

85. Since you saw the doctor have you talked about your visit to
    him with anyone?
    no   1
    yes
            spouse   2
            relative   3
            friend   4
            social worker   5
            other   6

86. Did he/she/they express any opinion about the consultation?
    yes:
            satisfied   1
            not satisfied (probe)   2
    no   3

87. Which of these phrases most nearly described your opinion of
    the consultation?
    very worthwhile   1
    worthwhile   2
    seemed a waste of time
            respondent's   3
            doctor's   4
    was a waste of time
            respondent's   5
            doctor's   6

Appendix 4 Consultation record.

Patient _____

Attendance (tick):   new/follow up

Patient's stated   (Underline which appear to be of most concern to
complaints/symptoms: patient.)

_____

_____

Procedures:
pulse	temperature	weight
bp	opthalmoscope	height
auriscope	other_____

Areas examined:
skin	locomotor system	abdomen/hernial
ears	eyes/nose	orifice
CNS	chest/heart	mouth/throat/tongue
rectal exam.	vaginal exam.	lymph glands
other _____

Result of   urine   bacteriology   histology
investigation: blood   x-ray   _____

Diagnosis:

1. _____ firm/provisional
                              prev/pres consultn.
                              given: yes/no

2. _____ firm/provisional
                              prev/pres consultn.
                              given: yes/no

3. _____ firm/provisional
                              prev/pres consultn.
                              given: yes/no

Action taken:
(a) Certificate issued: first/intermediate/final
(b) Prescription issued:
    (i) form _____ category _____
        condition _____ new/repeat
    (ii) form _____ category _____
        condition _____ new/repeat
    (iii) form _____ category _____
        condition _____ new/repeat
    (iv) form _____ category _____
        condition _____ new/repeat
(c) Advice/reassurance: _____

    _____

(d) Investigation:
        urine   bacteriology   histology
        blood   x-ray
        other (state) _____
(e) Referral: _____

    _____

(f) Follow-up: See again/discharge/return at own initiative

103

G.P.'s assessment of patient's reason(s) for attending:	(a) for certificate: first/intermediate/final
	(b) for prescription
	(c) for advice/reassurance re medical/social problem
	(d) for examination/investigation
	(e) result of investigation
	(f) for referral to specialist/within health team/social services
	(g) other _____
	(h) for check on progress
	(i) for diagnosis/confirmation of own diagnosis

Was patient justified in consulting?

Diagnosis 1	yes/no
Diagnosis 2	yes/no
Diagnosis 3	yes/no

How worried about problem/condition did patient appear to be?

Diagnosis 1	very/quite/not very/not at all
Diagnosis 2	very/quite/not very/not at all
Diagnosis 3	very/quite/not very/not at all

How worried do you consider it appropriate for this patient to be?

Diagnosis 1	very/quite/not very/not at all
Diagnosis 2	very/quite/not very/not at all
Diagnosis 3	very/quite/not very/not at all

How do you assess the seriousness of the patient's problem/ condition?

Medically:

Diagnosis 1	very/serious/quite/not
Diagnosis 2	very/serious/quite/not
Diagnosis 3	very/serious/quite/not

Socially:

Diagnosis 1	very/serious/quite/not
Diagnosis 2	very/serious/quite/not
Diagnosis 3	very/serious/quite/not

How well do you know the patient? Very well/quite well/not very well/not at all

Appendix 5 Questionnaire for Group B.

Year of b/sex: _____ 1 2   3 4   5 6   m/f

Registration: Dr. X/Y/other   <1 year 1–3 years 3–6 years 6–9 years 9 years+
                 1   2   3   1   2   3   4   5

Birth place: _____ 1   2   3   4   5

Res. U.K.: <1 year   1–5 years   6–10 years 10 years+   life
              1   2   3   4   5

Mar. status: single   married   widowed   sep.   div.
                1   2   3   4   5

Completed ed: 14   15   16   17   18   18+
                 1   2   3   4   5   6

Occupation: (prev. if retired) _____
               of husb. (prev. if decd.) _____
               1   2   3   4   5   6   7 (student)   8 (unemployed)

Religion: C/E RC J   JW CS Meth. Hdu. Mos. none
             1   2   3   4   5   6   7   8   9
             other _____ 11

104

1. When did you last consult a doctor at the practice?
   never   1
   <1 week   2
   1 week–1 month   3
   1 month–3 months   4
   3 months–6 months   5
   6 months–1 year   6
   1 year–2 years   7
   2 years+   8

2. Have you ever wanted to see the doctor before the earliest
   appointment offered to you?
   no   1
   don't remember   2
   first time attender   3
   yes: 4
         occasionally   1
         often   2
         not if urgent   3

3. How helpful do you find the receptionists when you are making
   an appointment?
   very helpful   1
   quite helpful   2
   receptionists vary   3
   don't know   4
   other (state)   5
   not helpful (probe)   6

4. If you had an appointment to see a particular doctor and found
   that the consultation was to be with another doctor, how would
   you feel about it?
   would not matter   1
   would depend on circumstances (probe)   2
   would not accept it (probe)   3
   would not like it (probe)   4
   other (state)   5

5. If you found that a medical student was to be present during a
   consultation with the doctor, how would you feel about it?
   would not mind   1
   would not like it (probe)   2
   would not like it in certain circumstances (probe)   3
   other (state)   4

6. If for some reason you did not want a medical student to be
   present during a consultation, would you ask the doctor to see
   you by yourself?
   yes   1
   don't know   2
   no (probe)   3

7. If you attended the surgery about a minor illness or injury would you, or would you not, be satisfied if a nurse attended to you instead of the doctor?

    yes   1
    don't know   2
    other (state)   3
    no (probe)   4

yes	1
don't know	2
other (state)	3
no (probe)	4

8. If you wanted to see a specialist and the present system was changed so that you could choose between going to him directly or going through your doctor, as we have to now, which would you prefer to do?

(a) prefer G.P. (probe)	1
(b) prefer specialist (probe)	2
don't know	3
(c) depends on circumstances (probe)	4
other (state)	5

9. Is there a doctor at the practice whom you think of as *your* doctor?

yes (probe)	1
no	2

10. How well do you think Dr. .... (given above) knows you?

very well	1
quite well	2
not very well	3
not at all	4
don't know	5
other (state)	6

11. Do you think your relationship with Dr. .... (given above) is (prompt)

impersonal and business-like	1
personal and friendly, or	2
business-like but friendly	3
don't know	4
other (state)	5

12. Do you think that talking to Dr. .... (given above) is (prompt)

always easy	1
sometimes difficult or	2
always difficult	3
don't know	4
other (state)	5

13. Why do you think that this is?

1. general dislike of doctors	1
2. doctor's manner	2
3. patient's difficulty in explaining	1
4. doctor too hurried	2
5. don't know	3
6. other (state)	4

14. Is there any other doctor whom you would prefer to see?
    yes (probe who/why/why has not changed)   1
    no   2
    don't know   3

15. Do you think that the doctor's interest in you should be (a) restricted to your medical condition, or that (b) he should also be interested in you as a person?
    (a)   1
    (b)   2
    don't know   3
    other (state)   4

16. From past experience of your doctor/doctors, do you think he does/they do take an interest in you as a person?
    yes   1
    don't know   2
    other (state)   3
    no (probe)   4

17. Which kind of doctor would you rather have (prompt)
    one who is impersonal and business-like   1
    one who is personal and friendly, or   2
    one who is business-like but friendly   3
    don't know   4

18. Do you ever feel nervous about seeing the doctor?
    never   1
    yes: 2
        always   1
        often   2
        occasionally   3

19. Why do you think this is?
    1. patient's temperament   1
    2. worried re possible outcome   2
    3. general dislike of seeing doctors   1
    4. manner of particular doctor   2
    5. don't know   3

20. If you had a serious personal problem which was depressing you and you wanted to talk to someone about it, who do you think you would turn to?
    spouse   1
    relation   2
    friend   3
    vicar/priest   4
    social worker   5
    tutor   6
    other   7
    would not turn to anyone   8
    would depend on circumstances   9
    don't know   11
    doctor (code 21/1)   12

21. Would you talk to your doctor about a personal problem or not?
        yes   1
        no   2
        don't know   3

23. If you saw the doctor about a troublesome condition would you, or would you not, want him to explain what the condition was?
        yes   1
        no   2
        would leave it to the doctor   3
        don't know   4
        other (state)   5

24. How full would you want his explanation to be?   1

25. From past experience of your doctor/doctors, how full do you think the explanation would be?   1

26. When the doctor gives you a prescription, do you or do you not, like him to tell you something about it?
        yes   1
        yes, if new to me   2
        would leave it to him to decide   3
        no   4
        don't know   5
        other (state)   6

27. What do you like to be told about a prescription?
        don't know   1
        1. name   2
        2. content   3
        3. form   4
        4. what it is for   1
        5. what effect it will have   2
        6. contra-indications   3
        7. how to take it   1
        other (state)   2

28. From past experience of your doctor/doctors, do you think you would be given this information or not?
        yes:
                all   1
                not all   2
                if one asks   3
        no   4
        depends on circumstances   5
        don't know   6

29. If the doctor were to arrange for you to have an investigation, e.g. an X-ray, or arrange for you to see someone else, would you want him to explain why it was necessary, or not?
        yes   1
        no   2
        would leave it to him   3
        don't know   4
        other (state)   5

108

30. From past experience of your doctor/doctors, do you think this would be explained to you, or not?

yes/probably	1
yes, if one asks	2
it would depend on circumstances	3
no	4
don't know	5
other (state)	6

31. If the doctor had not told you something you wanted to know during a consultation, do you think you would ask him about it or not?

yes	1
no	2
might	3
don't know	4
other (state)	5

32. Why do you think you might not ask him?   1
    * "Now I would just like to ask you a few questions about your general health."

33. Do you have any condition of illness which you have consulted the doctor about in the past but which you no longer expect him to help you with?

yes (probe)	1
no	2

34. Have you any condition or illness which you are continuing to see the doctor about?

yes (probe)	1
no	2

35. Would you describe this as a long term or a short term condition?

long term	1
short term	2
don't know	3
other (state)	4

36. How long have you been seeing the doctor about this?

<1 month	1
1 month–3 months	2
3 months–6 months	3
6 months–1 year	4
1 year–2 years	5
2 years–4 years	6
4 years+	7

37. Apart from this/During the past four weeks have you had any illness, injury, pain or discomfort which, you have not seen a doctor about?

yes (probe)	1
no	2
don't remember	3

38. Have you taken any action or treated the condition (given for 37) in any way?
>>> yes (probe + source of advice etc.)
>>>> a. medic.   1
>>>> b. non-medic.   2
>>>> c. self   3
>>>> d. chemist   4
>>> no   5

39. Can you say why you did not go to see the doctor about it?
>>> don't know   1
>>> other (state)   2

40. During the last four weeks have you suffered from (a) severe depression or tension, or from (b) *abnormal* tiredness, or (c) sleeplessness—*which you have not seen the doctor about*?
>>> yes:
>>>> a   1
>>>> b   2
>>>> c   3
>>> no   4

41. Are you still troubled by this?
>>> yes   1
>>> no   2

42. Have you had any advice about it from anyone?
>>> yes (probe)
>>>> a. medic.   1
>>>> b. non-medic.   2
>>>> a + b   3
>>> no   4

43. Did you follow this advice?
>>> yes   1
>>> no   2

44. Did the advice help with the .... (given for 40)?
>>> yes (in what way)   1
>>> no   2
>>> don't know   3

45. Apart from this/have you (a) taken any action or (b) treated the condition (given for 40) yourself?
>>> yes (probe)
>>>> a.   1
>>>> b.   2
>>>> a. + b.   3
>>> no   4

46. Do you think this helped?
>>> yes (probe)   1
>>> no   2
>>> don't know   3

47. Do you think your doctor would have been able to treat the condition .... (given for 40)?
>>> yes   1
>>> no (why not)   2
>>> don't know   3

48. Why did you not go to see him about it?

don't know	1
other	2
not a medical matter	3
not happy with doctor	4
not serious enough	1
felt able to treat it myself	2
too busy to see the doctor	3
don't like to bother the doctor	1
doctor too busy	2

49. Do you know what it was that may have caused the condition (given for 40)?

yes (probe)	1
respondent declined to answer	2
no	3

50. Do you think the doctor might have been able to help you with this/these problems (given for 49)?

yes	1
no (probe why not?)	2
don't know	3

51. Why did you not go to see him about it?

1. too busy to see the doctor	1
2. don't like to bother the doctor	2
3. did not think he would be sympathetic	3
4. not a medical matter	1
5. other (state)	2
don't know	3

Appendix 6.

Letter of initial contact for Group B.

Dear

My colleague and I are carrying out an enquiry into the National Health Service. We are particularly interested in the needs and expectations of patients in connection with their general practitioners. Your opinions in this matter are very important, as we are mainly concerned with the view of the patients, rather than that of the doctors.

We have discussed the objects of the enquiry with your doctor and he has supplied us with a list of his patients. From this list we have picked out at random a number of names, including yours, and we are now writing to ask if you will help us with our enquiry.

There is a slip attached to this letter which shows a suggested time and date for one of us to come and see you. If this is convenient, please tick the box provided. If the appointment is not convenient for you, please tick a box indicating one date and time when you would be able to see one of us. A stamped addressed envelope is enclosed for the return of the slip. We should be most grateful if you would post this back to us as soon as possible.

We feel sure that the results of the enquiry will be of value both to patients and th doctors. Thank you for your co-operation without which this project would not possible.

Yours sincerely,

Printed in Great Britain for Her Majesty's Stationery Office
By J. W. Arrowsmith Ltd., Bristol, BS3 2NT

Dd 597114 K20 7/79

THE DOCTOR/PATIENT RELATIONSHIP

RELATIONSHIP

A Study in General Practice

Freda Fitton, B.Sc., M.A. (Econ.),
Research Associate.

H. W. K. Acheson, O.B.E., M.B., Ch.B., F.R.C.G.P.,
Senior Lecturer.

Department of General Practice,
University of Manchester.

LONDON
HER MAJESTY'S STATIONERY OFFICE

The Research was sponsored by the Department of Health and Social Security.
The views expressed together with recommendations made are not necessarily those of the DHSS or any other Government Department.

ISBN 0 11 320685 2